At Your Fingertips

The Care & Maintenance of a Vagina.

ISBN   0-9629162-6-9

Printed in the U.S.A.

HYSTERIA PUBLICATIONS

is a small press dedicated to women's humor and social change. We publish a quarterly magazine, titled *Hysteria*, plus books, and calendars. We are always seeking work by women at our best and funniest. Please submit manuscripts, cartoons, art, and photographs to:

HYSTERIA PUBLICATIONS

Box 8581, Brewster Station
Bridgeport, CT 06605

Please include SASE and phone number with all submissions and allow six weeks for a reply.

Writers' guidelines for *Hysteria* are available with SASE.

This book was conceived by ...
Jerri Thomas

Nurtured by ...
Lysbeth Guillorn
Ellen Mayer
Ann Sussman

Brought to fruition by ...
Michele Ruschhaupt
Jennifer Sisca
Deborah Werksman

And showered with the gifts
of all the writers and cartoonists
in these pages ...

ABOUT THE WRITERS & CARTOONISTS

Josey Ballenger
is a New York City poet, writer, and book and music reviewer.

Alison Bechdel
is the creator of "Dykes To Watch Out For," a cartoon series published by Firebrand Press.

Donna Black
is a Texan, a freelance writer, and a regular contributor to Hysteria Magazine.

Andrea Carlisle
is the author of The Riverhouse Stories. She teaches creative writing at the Oregon Writers' Workshop.

Catherine Conant
is a Connecticut-based freelance writer and storyteller.

Cathy Crimmins
is a prolific humorist. Her eighth book, When My Parents Were My Age, will be published by Simon & Schuster in the spring of 1995. She lives in Philadelphia.

Diane Dimassa
is the creator of the quarterly comic-zine, Hothead Paisan — Homicidal Lesbian Terrorist.

Gyl Elliott
is a writer and Los Angeles civil servant. Her first novel is in progress.

Catherine Goggia
is a Chico, CA cartoonist.

Debra Gussman, M.D.
is a Denver, CO OB/GYN and creator of Personal Insights: A Self-Examination Kit for Women.

Nicole Hollander
is best known for her "Sylvia" comic strip, syndicated in 46 newspapers. Her 1995 feline astrology calendar, Under the Sign of the Cat, is published by Hysteria Publications.

Lisa Jansen
is a freelance writer living in Madison, WI.

Madeleine Begun Kane
is a writer, lawyer and oboe player. She lives in New York City.

Sheryl Kayne
is a Connecticut author and stand-up comic, and writes the syndicated column "The Weigh It Is".

Pamela Margoshes
is a freelance writer living in Washington D.C., who will soon be relocationg to Australia.

Jude McGee
is a radio and television host and producer, and is co-anchor of Feminist Analysis of the News on KPFK radio, Los Angeles.

Inga Muscio
writes a regular column called "Vagina Dentata" for Bluestocking, the unabashedly feminist publication.

Sara Nuss-Galles
writes fiction, memoirs and humor. Her children's book, Summer Detectives, is in search of a publisher.

Effin Older
is a Vermont writer and photographer. Her book, Horseradish and Apple Pie, is to be published in 1995 by Harcourt Brace.

Nina Paley

is a San Francisco Bay Area cartoonist and creator of "Nina's Adventures".

Rina Piccolo

is a Toronto cartoonist featured in many comic anthologies.

Stephanie Piro

is a New Hampshire cartoonist. Her first book, Men! Ha! is published by Laugh Lines Press.

Libby Reid

lives in New York City has several collections of her cartoons in print.

Laura Allen Sandhu

is at work on her dissertation on African diaspora poetry. She lives in Tracy, CA.

Dorothy Shiels

is a freelance writer living in Rhode Island. She specializes in humorous travel articles.

Nina Silver

writes on feminism and metaphysics. Her volume of poetry, Birthing, will be published in 1995 by Woman in the Moon.

Maureen Stanton

is a freelance writer in Portland, ME.

Mary-Lou Weisman

is a writer, journalist and humorous essayist. Her satirical book on middle age will be published in Spring 1995 by Workman Publishing Co.

Leslie What

is a freelance writer with a forthcoming piece, "Compatability Clause" in Fantasy and Fiction magazine.

CONTENTS

CALLING *IT* WHAT IT *IS*

SURROUNDING MENSTRUATION

THE SEXUAL COMPONENT

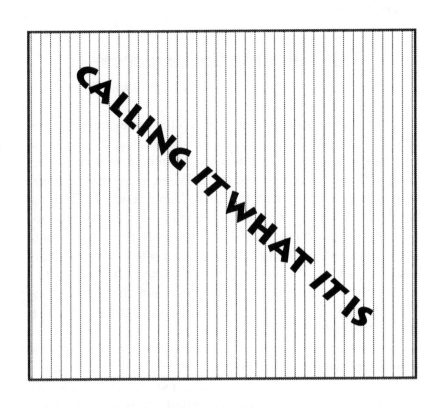

CALLING IT WHAT IT IS

Truth and the Consequences
by Donna Black

Menstruation by Many Other Names
by Sheryl Kayne

Whatever Happened to Vagina Envy?
by Sara Nuss-Galles

What IS a Douche Bag?
by Laura Allen Sandhu

Truth and the Consequences

by Donna Black

I'm constantly amazed at how many other names are used to re-fer to the vagina or the penis, especially when dealing with children. For example, we were at a restaurant with another family when their little girl turned to her mom and stated, "Mommy, my she-she needs to go wee-wee." And with the usual chain reaction, her brother piped up, "Daddy, my he-he needs to go pee-pee." Fortunately, be-cause my two girls had no idea what their friends were talking about, I didn't have to face the nightmare of taking a toddler to a foreign bathroom. On another occasion, while playing at the park, I actu-ally heard a man say to his son who was holding his crotch, "Hey Tim, my man, do ya need to go drain your tool (grunt, grunt)?" I mean, come on — his "tool"?

She-she, he-he, and tool? Nope, I decided that when my girls were old enough to ask, they would simply be told the real names of the body part and bodily function in question. So, when my 3 1/2-year-old pointed below her waist and asked why water came out, I explained that it was called a vagina and the water was called urine and please not to drink it or try to get her little sister to drink it. And when she happened to see her dad using the bathroom and asked what that thing was and why he stood up, I simply told her that that "thing" was a penis and that's what men and boys used to urinate (and please not to grab it like a rope to swing from ever again ....)

For awhile she was saying, "Daddy has a peanut," and because I didn't want my child accidently to create yet another ridiculous slang word for penis (not to mention my husband's embarrassment over being called the man with the peanut), I spent quite a bit of time getting her to pronounce penis correctly.

Alas, sometimes complete honesty can backfire, and even though I'm still a firm believer in teaching kids the real words for any part of the body and its functions, I'm quite sure our "straight talk" was not appreciated during our most recent journey to Hot Springs Village, Arkansas.

Usually we go there to visit relatives; this time the trip was due to the death of Uncle Tom. We hadn't wanted to take the kids, but Aunt Betty had insisted that they would be "rays of sunshine" during an otherwise somber event. It seemed Aunt Betty was right, too. All the people we met (90% of them were over the age of 70) seemed to enjoy watching the antics of our two little girls. Even during the memorial service, the girls behaved admirably. In fact, by the time the service was over, I was in a blissful and euphoric state, knowing I had two of the best children in the world.

Then came the dinner following the memorial service. Because everyone just loved our little darlings (my youngest was blowing kisses to everyone), the table we chose soon filled up with grandmas, grandpas, and great-grandparents eager to spend more time with our two girls.

So there we all were, my husband and I beaming with pride over our perfect children, surrounded by elders anxiously waiting to hear what lovable statements the two little angels would make. Well, the oldest angel decided not to waste this moment in the spotlight and with a glance around the entire table, she took a deep breath and began pointing to each of our table mates while saying clearly and loudly (oh, so clearly and loudly): "You have a penis and you have a vagina and you have a penis and you have a vagina and you have a penis and you have a vagina and ...." until all the vaginas and penises at our table had been addressed.

I had never before seen the domino effect of mouths dropping open in shock and, quite frankly, I hope never to again. All I could think during those moments of great trial and tribulation (with my husband muttering, "You just had to teach her to say penis correctly, didn't you ....") was that at least my littlest angel hadn't let me down. As I bent my head to kiss her silky soft blond halo, I couldn't help but notice (as did everyone else) that she was quite busy with her finger up her nose ...

❖

Menstruation by Many Other Names

by Sheryl Kayne

I remember it well. I was only 11 years old and my parents were out of town. I think they were visiting my grandmother in New Jersey. My girlfriend Donna and I were listening to music in my room when I swung my legs around to change position. She saw red.

"The flag's up. You've got the curse," she squealed.

We ran into the bathroom where I examined my condition.

I called my mother to announce my badge of honor. "*Mazel tov!*" said Mom. "You've got your friend! There are sanitary pads in the bottom of my bathroom closet."

That was the first and last conversation my mother and I had about my period. I decided to do a better job with my own two daughters. I started planning it all out soon after they were born. I collected books with titles like *Period* and *When the Egg Breaks*. I committed myself to fulfilling my matriarchal responsibility to properly educate and fully inform my offspring.

Monthly, I discussed with them what was happening with me. "Mommy is menstruating. A menstrual cycle is normal. Mommy's onset of menses was at age 11. You will probably be around that same age when you experience the monthly discharge of blood, secretions, and tissue debris from the uterus that recurs monthly in nonpregnant, breeding-age primate females. Menstruation is the readjustment of the uterus to the nonpregnant state following proliferative changes accompanying ovulation."

My lovely daughters matured under my watchful eye. One fateful, dreary, rainy, cold day in October, I sent my little girl of only 10 years and seven months of age off to school. She called at 10:30 a.m. "I got IT, Mom. I asked the school nurse if I could go on the stick, but she didn't have any, so I'm on the rag."

I answered, "*Mazel tov.*"

❖

Whatever Happened to Vagina Envy?

by Sara Nuss-Galles

Penis "the copulatory organ of the male of a higher vertebrate animal that, in mammals, usually provides also the channel by which urine leaves the body and is typically a cylindrical organ ...." blah, blah, blah. By the time I've read this, not only am I confused, but I'm losing interest. And I wish someone could explain to me why there is no picture. Right in the next column there's a sketch of a pen holder. Is Webster saying it's more important to know what a pen holder looks like than a penis? What about those of us who might get the two confused? Who makes stupid decisions like this? And why does every word I look up give me three other words to look up?

I am sitting in the Alessandro Volta Elementary School library going through *Webster's Unabridged Dictionary*. I'm supposed to be researching early explorers, but somehow I got sidetracked. I'm very disappointed by the lack of hard information on penis. My eyes go to the next entry: *Penis envy*.

It says, "the unverbalized longing of a girl or woman to be a boy or man." Huh? That doesn't sound like anything I've ever felt. Is this some kind of joke? And, not surprising, there's no picture of penis envy, either.

It's 10 minutes into 6th period, and it's obvious that I have my work cut out for me. I'm twelve years old, a remarkably curious lover of words — especially certain mysterious, sexy words. And now, I'm desperately seeking the boy thing that would be what penis envy is to a girl. Copulatory, one of the words I have to look up from the penis entry, can wait.

From my experience with two older brothers and a father, all of whom walk around the house in saggy boxer shorts, I understand that penis is to boy what vagina is to girl. So, vagina envy it must be, and I flip pages to the v's.

Here it is. *Vagina*: "a canal that leads from the uterus of a female mammal to the external orifice of the genital canal." I'm provided with no basis for vaginal comparison, as this word also has no picture. On the facing page, however, there is a nice line drawing of a valet. Well, if I ever have a valet, I'll be able to compare it to the picture in the dictionary.

Meanwhile, I skim the column to *vaginal process*, then *vaginal smear* (I can't believe they put in such a disgusting thing, whatever it is). I glance back up to where *vagina envy* should be. It's not there! How can this be? Puzzled, I raise my head and glance around the library. The librarian spots me and stage-whispers across the room, "Need help, Sara?" She knows me by name because I spend a lot of time taking out books and, especially, using the dictionary.

"Uh uh," I whisper back, feeling the heat rise in my face and quickly turning the page in case she comes over.

Clearly, I've chosen the wrong phrase. But what else could be the opposite of penis envy? Nipple envy, breast envy? Even I realize that this doesn't make sense, because men have those as well as women, so what's to envy? What could be the word for boys who long to be girls? Whom can I ask? How can I find out?

Okay. Time is flying. I'll ponder this later in health class or geography. But, right now, while I've got this unabridged dictionary .... I turn back to *copulation*, which I've never heard of before. It says, "to join or unite ... " — boring! But then, "to unite in sexual intercourse: engage in coitus." Again, no pictures, and two more words to look up. Since I'm already in the c's, I'll start with coitus, a word that can't be much since I've never seen it scrawled anywhere.

There's a very stupid drawing of a coil, and right next to that is *coitus*, a word I can't figure out how to pronounce. How many syllables can one short word have? It says, "the physical union of male and female genitalia ..." (another word to look up), "accompanied by ..." now it gets interesting — "rhythmic movements leading to the ejaculation ...;" here we go again. I wish

I could risk writing these words down so I could remember what to look up next.) " ... of semen from the penis into the female reproductive tract; also: intercourse." Aha!

After that, I'm too flustered for *orgasm*, as a consequence of which I spend the next 20 years trying to define exactly what it is.

Fortunately, the bell soon rings, signaling the end of 6th, and our library period is over. I get into line, clutching my sweaty, but blank, sheet of five-ring notebook paper. I still have a report due on Ponce de Leon, whom I associate with penis envy for the rest of my life.

As I head back to homeroom, I decide to change topics. Suddenly, I feel an affinity with the letter v, and the explorer Vasco da Gama pops into my head. So, Vasco, whom I fondly nickname "vagina envy," becomes the subject of my paper, and the seeker to whom I dedicate my ongoing linguistic exploration.

❖

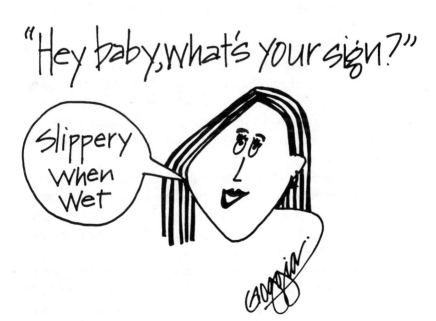

Cartoon by Catherine Goggia

What IS a Douchebag?

by Laura Allen Sandhu

I am on a campaign. An academic way to state my purpose would be: Demystifying and Revaluing Female Body Experience. A better way to get it across might be to simply ask, "What IS a douche bag, anyway? Why is it an insult to be called one? And why do you never see one lying on somebody's coffee table?"

Sure, bodily functions are generally kept hush-hush, for men and women alike. But there is an undeniable double standard where female functions are concerned. They are so taboo that even a box of maxipads doesn't have the word MENSTRUAL prominently emblazoned across the front. It's a "feminine hygiene" product. Imagine a drugstore with a sign along one wall: Menstrual Bleeding Products. Half the store would become a deserted wasteland; people would shield their eyes and the eyes of their children as they trekked past the dreadful words on their way to the Dr. Scholl's foot care department.

One euphemism that really bugs me is "feminine itching." It conjures up the image of a delicate woman tastefully dressed in flowing white, crossing her legs and almost imperceptibly squirming with vague discomfort (although you will never even see a squirm in an advertisement). Exactly which aspect of her femininity is itching we are not to know. Something hidden and mysterious, perhaps her fallopian tubes.

Now compare this to the male equivalent, which is not given a sissy name like "masculine inflammation," but is spelled out in rough, tough, four-letter words: JOCK ITCH. Immediately you have visions of locker rooms filled with hairy, smelly men brazenly scratching their sweaty crotches.

Of course, much of what goes on in the female anatomy has no male equivalent. Like douching, a practice that has thoroughly mystified me since early girlhood. I saw commercials that spoke with a knowing look about "freshness," and I surreptitiously scanned douche packages in the drugstore. These were not at all helpful. In a bathroom closet at a friend's house, I thought I saw a douche bag the size of my grandmother's largest hot water bottle. Of course, it could have been an enema bag, but in either case, the same two questions apply: Where does all that water *go*? And how does it get back *out*?

Do you have to hold it in there the way you do when you gargle or do you have to stand on your head? I pictured it leaking out a little at a time all day long, like those devices my mom would buy to water the houseplants while we were on vacation, and that didn't sound "fresh" at all to me.

I still turn these questions over in my mind when I see one of those TV ads where a mother counsels her daughter in the vague euphemistic dialect of douchespeak, and the daughter miraculously understands, pulling a Summer's Eve box out of her purse with a wink. And I wonder how the women acting in the commercial — and the men (most likely) filming and directing it — can bear to coexist for an entire workday with the big, unspoken, unspeakable, inexplicable word DOUCHE hanging in the air over their heads.

Next question: Is there a link between feminine deodorant suppositories and those new plug-in-the-wall dissolving air fresheners?

> **"Excuse me, everybody,
> I have to go to the bathroom.
> I really have to telephone,
> but I'm too embarrassed to say so."**
> Dorothy Parker,
> from the *Beacon Book of Quotations by Women*,
> compiled by Rosalie Maggio

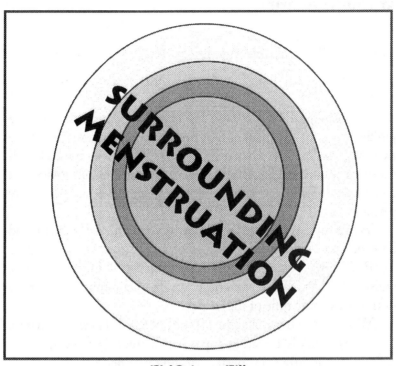

PMS-in-a-Pill
by Pamela Margoshes

Give Me Chocolate. Period.
by Sheryl Kayne

For My Daughter
by Catherine Conant

(One Up) For Les Menses
by Josey Ballenger

Vaginal Fashion: What's In and Out
by Cathy Crimmins

How To Mummify Your Used Sanitary Pads
by Leslie What

That Not-So-Often Talked About Subject
by Maureen Stanton

PMS-in-a-Pill

by Pamela Margoshes

I *like* having PMS. Maybe I'm crazy, some kind of hormone junkie, living for the thrill of that first crescendo of emotion, those first pings and pangs of radiating anxiety. But I've come to cherish those great bursts of anger, irritation, and intensified creativity that come every month and last for about a week and a half before my period.

While mine is admittedly a minority opinion, it's one that could become more widespread.

PMS gives a woman a perfect excuse for all kinds of wacky, antisocial behaviors that she'd never dream of committing at a more hormonally static time of the month.

While in the hormonal throttle of PMS, I feel perfectly free to:

a) honk like mad at any driver who deviates even slightly from perfect driving practices;

b) sink into a heap at any time and anywhere and let loose with moans and groans of the most shocking and sensual nature.

For manic persons like me, PMS is the hormonal equivalent of a papal dispensation. I get to act even more maniacally than usual and blame any of my weirder actions — like breaking into loud birdlike noises in public or making sudden, unanticipated break-dance movements — on hormonal hegemony.

And I feel so creative and so energetic that I can get the entire house cleaned in one hormone-propelled hour.

I know that PMS has gotten really bad press, that it's not generally regarded as a condition to aspire to, or to look forward to with glee.

But I look at it this way: Since I know that it's inevitable, that it's as entrenched in me as, say, lust or greed, there has to be an up side to it. Not that I credit Nature with such enlightened teleology, but it's in *my* nature to be perverse. If everyone else hates something, then I like it.

PMS allows me to make such normally out-of-the-socially-acceptable-sphere comments as "I've got to rush home: I don't want to miss *Full House*."

I've come to appreciate the roller-coaster ride of being female. I'm a feminist with a phenomenal appreciation for my monthly wild ride.

I think we live in truly glorious times now. Women have the right to either cherish or curse their hormones. After years and years of cursing my hormones and dreading those 10 days before menstruation, I welcome them now.

It's a time of intensified personality, of full-speed-ahead creativity, and of manic bouts of energy and bravado (yes, with terrible lows, too, but the highs more than compensate). A time of awe over the power of my body and its processes.

I wouldn't be surprised if one day it's actually medically proven that PMS is an excellent creativity stimulator, and that artists and writers (and dedicated housekeepers) do indeed profit imaginatively from those days of tumult and frenzy before menstruation.

I, who used to spend my PMS days in a fog of massive doses of ibuprofen, now say: *Let the good (hormonal) times roll!*

I revel in it now. I say what the hell!

Bring on the anxiety and the pains in the womb and the swollen breasts and the temporary five pounds of water gain.

It's all worth it, because last month, in an extended bout of prostaglandin fervor, I wrote the first chapter of my new novel.

And two months ago, I woke up in the middle of the night and rewrote the theory of relativity. This month, I figure I'll take on the theory of chaos.

Of course, PMS does bring on an occasional night of supreme delusions — but what's a few nights of thinking you're Cher if you're able to solve the kind of philosophical problems that bedeviled

Schopenhauer, Jean-Paul Sartre, and Barbara Cartland. *Plus* clean behind the oven.

I'm convinced that in the 21st century, when PMS is finally given its creative and medical due, *everyone* will want it.

There will be PMS-in-a-pill for anyone who wants a seven- to 10-day stretch of philosophical invincibility (coupled with the ability to cry — oh, so gratifyingly — for six hours straight). Folks will scarf it down like candy.

❖

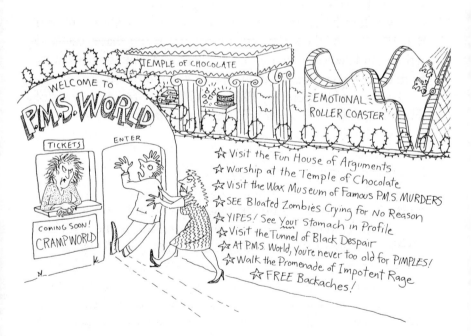

Cartoon by Libby Reid, from *Do You Hate Your Hips More Than Nuclear War?* (Penguin Books)

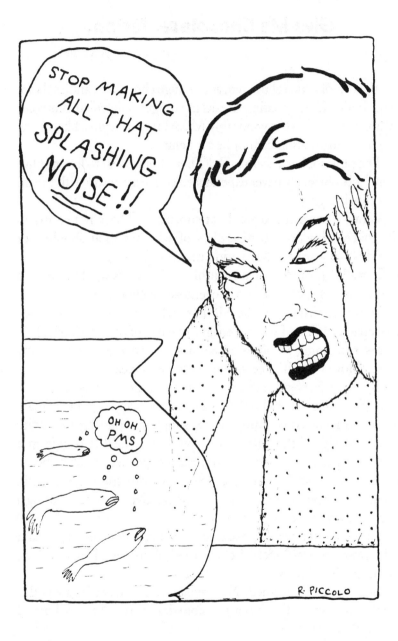

Cartoon by Rina Piccolo, from *Stand Back, I Think I'm Gonna Laugh* (Laugh Lines Press)

Give Me Chocolate. Period.

by Sheryl Kayne

Visions of little yellow, red, and orange chocolate candies dance on my brain. Green coating streaks my tongue. Chocolate bits color my fingernails. Once my monthly M&M frenzy begins, I know the onset of menstruation cannot be far behind.

The philosopher Cicero said: "Thou shouldst eat to live, not live to eat." He obviously never experienced coffee ice cream with Heath Bar crunch.

When I crave chocolate, I eat chocolate. That's not eating to live, that's living to eat; regardless of whether thou shouldst or shouldnst, I havest to: My period maketh me do it.

It is all part of that great monthly cycle, as it is written from up above: Once a month, you will overdose on chocolate.

Nothing satisfies me like M&Ms. Maybe it's because they are so poppable. When I was a teenager, one bag of plain M&Ms, 1.69 ounces, containing 54 bite-size candies, was enough to quench my desire. However, with age, my appetite has increased.

Today, at forty-something, I need a one-pound bag to get me through. There are 400 M&Ms in the pounder bag. Hallelujah. What a bargain. By counting out my supply and putting 50 candies in each of eight little baggies and placing each little baggie in a necessary place — coat pocket, slacks pocket, pocket book, refrigerator top shelf, desk top, glove compartment, reading chair, and under my pillow — I consume one M&M at a time, creating a time-released effect.

I used to feel guilty, ashamed, lustful, sinful, obsessed and embarrassed by my M&M frenzy. Even abnormal. I tried to hide it from my loved ones.

But I've been redeemed. New research on food cravings says this is my body's way of filling a physiological need. See? I knew I needed those M&Ms.

Chocolate contains caffeine, theobromine, fat, and calories, all in a delicious combination, I might add. When I eat chocolate, endorphins are released in my brain, making me feel just as good as if I had run a mile. This way I save on stress to my knees and sweat on my socks.

And, anyway, I have no choice. If I don't eat my M&Ms, my period might not come.

For My Daughter

by Catherine Conant

I like to browse through antiques and junk shops — the junkier the better. More often than not, I am drawn toward those pieces of flotsam that are less a valuable collectible than a tangible link to an individual I will never know. Possessing something that was once important to a forgotten person fulfills a curious need to place myself in the past.

One day, in the time before I had children, I found a small china cup in a shop. It is as thin as an eggshell, is rimmed with gold, and has an oval wreath of pastel flowers. In the center of the oval, written with flowing, golden script are the words, "To my daughter." It is Victorian sentiment at its most charming; and so I took it home and put it on a shelf and told it to wait. For what, I was not exactly sure.

Later, with as much anticipation and joy as any child deserves, my children were born. My son first, and then my daughter. And still the cup sat on the shelf.

Even more time has passed, and now I look at my daughter, with her body poised on the edge of puberty and womanhood, and I have made a decision.

When I was at the age she is now, I was tightly budded, all angles and bones, angry with those I called prissy girls. With their carefully matched sportswear and their secret glances, they were knowledgeable in subjects I scarcely knew existed. They swept past me like royalty, scorning their membership in the old neighborhood gang for more important meetings. I was furious and I was uneasy.

My mother, for all her love and attention, simply could not bring herself to discuss menstruation. She had made vague mention of difficult times ahead, but I responded to her unspoken limits and asked no questions. The blue booklet with the mysterious coded message "Moddess ... because" appeared, and just as suddenly, vanished. One day, after discovering a box of Kotex hidden in the closet, I shredded them all, convinced that something valuable must be tucked inside each one, so carefully were they wrapped. Mother didn't say anything; I followed her cue.

When, suddenly, on a hot July day I discovered I was bleeding without visible wounds, I ran, panicked, into the house. Wordlessly, she showed me how to rig my harness, roll up the evidence in yards of toilet paper, and hide it in the bottom of the wastebasket. Most of all, she spoke sadly of limits, of cautions, and reminded me not to let anyone know.

How could they not know, I wondered? She had fixed me up with one of those cumbersome bundles that caused me to walk with a rolling gait, like some sailor newly returned to shore. Where moments before I climbed the fences with my brothers, now I perched on the edge of a bench, and tried to figure out how to sit on the thing. I was set apart, frightened, and confused. Suddenly I was different from my friends, yet I didn't want to be like the other girls I knew. I was lost, my sense of identity buried in layers of cotton, unfit to be seen, not to be discussed.

That will not happen to my daughter.

Already, she has heard whispers from her friends. She has come home and spoken about this with a mixture of dread and fascination, having heard words that make her uneasy: Blood, pain, curse. I will shield her from the attitude that I know can strip her of her sense of well-being and leave her feeling betrayed by her body.

She knows the technical information, but the connection, the perspective by which she will always this aspect of her female being, is mine to shape.

And so we will celebrate. She already knows when the time comes, we will embrace it with ritual. Part of me envies her her sense of anticipation, her unshadowed willingness to enter this new phase of her life, but then motherhood is often sweetest when old wounds are soothed by the balm of better choices.

If school is in session, she may take the day off. We will go shopping, buy new clothes, go to the movies. She may have a new haircut if she so desires. We will tell her father and her brother and they will congratulate her, and we will prepare a special dinner. She will enter into this most powerful moment of girl made woman knowing, truly, that her menstrual period is not a thing to loathe or rail against. She will accept from the onset what I struggled for years to understand: that it is the cyclical reaffirmation of her womanhood and, as such, it should be honored.

And then I will give her the cup.

(One Up) For Les Menses

by Josey Ballenger

My loony, lunar friend —
disheveled and quirky in appearance
but downright serious in manner —
arrives at the most inappropriate of times
(When isn't it?),
Without invitation or explanation,
she draws attention to herself in various shades of red,
just rushing, gushing, up when I meet with my
boss/client/lover/friend/some other person I want to impress.

Despite her lack of manners
(she doesn't forewarn me —
and not even after years of experience can I predict precisely her arrival —
nor does she apologize),
she insists she is not only summoned but on schedule;
despite the midnight drugstore runs I make to clean up after her
and her bloating, cramping, gaseous consorts;
despite her taking over the bathroom,
ruining my clothes,
and spilling onto my bed...

Despite the panic, the pain, the rush, the mess,
the trouble and the expense,
I welcome her six-day stays;
indeed, I worry when she doesn't show up.

She comes whimsically but naturally,
rather than in a "regular" but half-assed, man-made form,
reminding me of what I am,
and what I can be.

Vaginal Fashion: What's In and Out

by Cathy Crimmins

I don't know when I first began thinking about how dull vaginal fashion has become. Maybe it was a couple of years ago, when a painter friend who'd always wanted to do a still life titled "Tampax Box on Toilet Back" called to give me the bad news. "They've got new boxes," she sobbed into the phone. "Those horrible little tasteful white flowers are gone. The new ones look like the cover of a corporate annual report, *and when you take off the cellophane, it says 'Tampax' right on the box!*"

She refused to be comforted, even when I pointed out how she'd hated the hypocrisy behind the old Tampax box of 40 — the way it was meant to look like it really wasn't filled with tampons, when everyone who went into your bathroom knew damn well what was in the blue box. Meanwhile, I craved sympathy for my own fashion loss, the "junior tampon," which I hear is coming back, but which I can never find.

There are no more euphemisms in the world of vaginal fashion. In these post-Toxic Shock times I bleed into Mega-Ultra-Maxi-Mini pads and medically-sanctioned tampons "designed by a woman gynecologist," not quaint old napkins. But I kind of miss the less enlightened days, when you could read a full-page ad for a feminine hygiene product without having the faintest idea of how it fit into any orifice of your body. In the true sense of fashion, the old-style packaging decorated with flowers and butterflies and pink lace provided the delusion I needed to go on.

The decidedly functional emphasis in women's hygiene gadgets these days is kind of depressing. Other common sanitary products at least show design flair. Huggies makes Disney diapers. Even adhesive bandages, which are not, after all, that far in function from the subject at hand, have cartoon pictures on them. By contrast, the designers of intimate objects for women lag sadly behind. There's my diaphragm case, for example. For years the rubber saucers came in a bland, pure white casing. But the latest one, an attempt at an updated look, is a hideous beige thing that seems hopelessly dated, like an avocado refrigerator. Not something I'd choose to have lying around on my bedside table even though it ends up there all the time. I'd definitely pay a few bucks extra for rhinestones or velvet or a picture of Mickey Mouse to match my bedroom decor. For that matter, maybe the designers could work on the diaphragm itself. We already have condoms in neon colors.

But let me stop beating around the bush, as so many manufacturers of fem-hygiene products have done for years. Why don't they have pictures of girls throwing coffee cups at their husbands and boyfriends, or clutching their abdomens in agony? Ads for headache and indigestion-related products show people grimacing or holding their heads. What's currently on the drugstore shelves is more notable for its amusement quotient than its aesthetic value or integrity: Kimberly-Clark's New Freedom pads, for example show a woman in sensible khaki hiking pants jumping up for joy. Did she just get her period, or buy a Toyota? And the best that tampon marketers seem able to do is o.b.'s much vaunted ad line — the things really were designed by a real, live, woman gynecologist — Dr. Judith Esser, from West Germany. In fact, they are even manufactured in Deutschland, which makes them the BMW of vaginal fashion. Now there's a status marketing angle that's been overlooked.

Finally, I've discovered that romance in women's product packaging still lurks in the douche section, which seems to have been caught in a time warp in about 1965. The boxes are amusing enough to make me want to douche someday.

I think we've been getting the short end of the string when it comes to fashion for the vagina because it's still not considered polite for girls to take much interest in the insertion of inanimate objects. I say it's time that feminine functions received equal rights. All you designers out there: take note.

How to Mummify Your Used Sanitary Pads

by Leslie What

I learned these techniques in junior high; they would probably need to be modified today. Things were different then: Kennedy was president; candy bars cost only 10 cents; we used pads instead of tampons; and toilet paper came in unperforated rolls. Still, perhaps the lessons of my youth, like the mummies of old, should be preserved.

The order to mummify came after the janitor, a slow-thinking man named Earl Schoom, happened upon a soiled sanitary napkin in one of those white revolving-door napkin bins that used to be on the floors of girls' bathrooms. My friend Cyndi, who was sneaking a cigarette in another stall, saw it happen. Earl Schoom had lifted off the revolving-door top and was grabbing handfuls of gum wrappers and trash to put into his large garbage can, when he touched a soiled napkin with his bare hands. On most days, Earl Schoom looked a lot like an unpeeled, boiled potato. But that one day, he picked up the pad, held it out in front of him as if he were holding a bloody tapeworm, and ran screaming across campus to the principal's office. Earl Schoom had become a wild man.

The sanitary napkin, growing more and more unsanitary by the hour, was placed in a display case as a grim reminder of the cost of carelessness.

"Disgusting to put a man through that," our gym teacher Miss Plink lectured the next day. Especially a man like Earl Schoom, who could not understand such things. Every girl, guilty or not, had been felled by shame.

One day during track, Miss Plink blew her whistle and called the girls to stand in a straight line just behind the sand pit. Miss Plink was a tall, thin woman who looked like a butter knife with fork tines for legs. She was way too tan, even for a Southern Californian, and her skin was the texture and color of a football, which none of us girls had ever been allowed to play. At her side was a large brown bag.

"I've been asked to demonstrate," she began. She took a box of sanitary napkins from the bag, opened it, and removed one clean pad that she held out in front of her. "Exhibit A," she said. Cyndi, standing beside me, snickered. Miss Plink blew her whistle again — so loudly that everyone's ears rang.

"You think this is funny," she said. "Well, think about what it would feel like if your father found your bloodied sanitary napkin in the trash?" Her eyes narrowed. "Or worse, what if your best friend's brother found your used sanitary napkin and showed it to all his friends?"

No one could argue with that, especially me. Cyndi had a brother who would have given up everything to embarrass me.

Next, Miss Plink took a roll of toilet paper from her bag. "Exhibit B," she said. She carefully folded the sanitary pad onto itself. She used the same fold we had learned in origami.

She started the roll, then wound half the roll of toilet paper around the sanitary pad, making quarter turns from time to time to cover it completely. When she had finished, the mummified pad was the size of a diaper.

"Now, let's practice," she said, and no one dared to challenge her. "We'll take turns," she said. "They only gave me one roll of toilet tissue for all of you."

Exactly 29 days later, Earl Schoom was seen running and screaming through the school, followed by a 50-foot white tapeworm. He ran into the parking lot and was never heard from again.

Miss Plink said nothing about it, but I heard from Cyndi, who had been sneaking cigarettes in another stall, that Earl Schoom had been cleaning the girls' rest room as usual. He had emptied the trash and had seen something wrapped inside a thousand layers of toilet tissue. He had patiently and methodically unwrapped his booty, expecting to find riches, no doubt. Yet what he found was a bloodied pad that moistened his fingertips and made the toilet tissue stick to them.

Not long after that, the white revolving-door napkin bins were lined with paper bags that could be removed without viewing the contents. I continued to mummify my used pads at school, but when I tried it at home, my mother told me to stop. "You're using too much toilet paper," was all she said.

❖

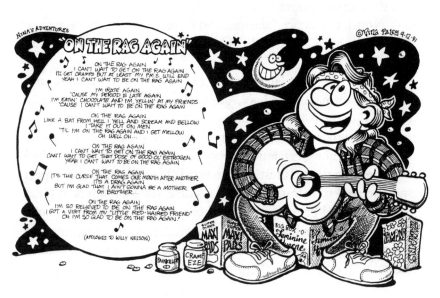

Cartoon by Nina Paley

That Not So Often Talked About Subject

by Maureen Stanton

A friend of mine once said, "I get philosophical when I bleed." She wasn't talking about a paper cut. So this month, while bleeding, I got philosophical *about* bleeding.

I grew up in the era when sex education was disguised as filmstrips of Netsilik Eskimos. This may have been a large step for womanhood compared to the previous generation, but it was a far cry from pedagogy. Because of this menstrual information blackout, I feel compelled to write about this subject. Also, because nobody else writes about it.

They don't talk about it either. I tried to make a PMS joke in a mixed crowd. Perhaps the staff meeting wasn't exactly the place for such a joke, but, hey, everyone: Ease up! There's certainly no need to keep menstruation in the closet. In reality, a woman would be more likely to say, "I'm flowing like the Mississippi," than "Did you ever get that not-so-fresh feeling?"

Things have changed though, and today we have tampon commercials on television, and in prime time. I guess it's about time to tell children what all those pink plastic tubes are that they find on the beach and use to build sand castles. A friend and I once counted 18 pink plastic tampon tubes from our blanket to the water at a beach in Massachusetts. It was a sort of modern-day Hansel and Gretel trail, but instead of leading to the horrible witch's gingerbread home, the pink trail markers led to the horrible humans' sewage depository — the ocean. At least we found our way back to the blanket okay.

Information about the necessities of womanhood were not always so publicly known. My first devastating experience with menstruation came when I was just eight years old. I was perched upon the porcelain throne, legs dangling, when I spied an interesting waxy blue bag in the waste basket. Upon opening it, to my horror, I discovered a huge, blood-soaked, white gauzelike bandage-type thing. I didn't have a word for it back then, but I knew it was serious. I rushed to my mother. "Mom, who was hurt?" "No one," she said, but I showed her the bloody evidence, to which she replied, "No one. Now put that back and don't go nosing through the wastebasket. Just you mind your own business." That incident left me permanently scarred, so just for that, I am writing this article (in extremely poor taste) to mortify my mother, and Ma, I'm using my *real name.* But at least I was not out in left field like my roommate Elaine.

For years she thought those things were to put in your shoes to cushion your feet. To give her some credit, she did begin to get suspicious when she noticed there weren't any in her father's closet. After all, her father was the one with the bunions.

Years later, my mother had one of my sisters call me in from playing ("Mom wants to talk to you" — never a good sign), and as I sat in an inner tube and watched her iron in our basement, she divined that *that* should be the moment of my womanly enlightenment. She gave me "the talk." Soon after, I was outfitted with the menstrual apparatus, the specially designed pad-friendly underwear, and the menstrual garter-belt-like thing, both meant to hold a bulky wadola of cotton/fiber/chemicals/unknown other materials between my skinny 12-year-old-legs without the world noticing.

Then, the day came. I was in sixth grade, at the school bookstore during recess, when I experienced excruciating abdominal pain. I was certain I was dying of food poisoning and lay on the floor to do just that. I managed to survive the rest of the day, and the rest of sixth grade, but I was a changed person. I was a WOMAN.

My mother betrayed me that day. She told my father. I was downstairs watching *Gilligan's Island* (I remember so clearly — one of the headhunter episodes), when my father, in front of all my siblings, said, "Congratulations. I heard you became a woman today." Aaaaaaaaaaaaaahhhhhh! I ran upstairs screaming, "Mom, why did you tell him?"

This experience wasn't as bad as Wendy's, whose menses first visited her at school, during lunch, all over her seat. She was taken to the nurse's office, but within seconds, the entire seventh grade knew, and filed past the besmirched chair. As for Wendy, well, she joined the debate team.

I have my own menstrual horror story, though, to pass on to my progeny. I read on the back of the box of mini-pads that they could be worn at all times, even during swimming. So, confidently, I affixed one to the crotch of my bathing suit during swim team practice. During the warm-up laps I felt the mini-pad detach and slowly creep up the back of my bathing suit like an alien life-form, and I knew, I knew, that sooner or later that thing was going to pop out and rise to the surface of the water, forever placing me in that small group of people who can never, ever again lead a normal teenhood because of some irreparably embarrassing incident (read: with Wendy on the debate team). But I saw my chance, between laps. I got out of the pool and edged my way back to the surrounding chain-link fence. I reached down my back into my bathing suit and grabbed the renegade mini-pad, bunching it up in my fist. Then I squatted down, pretended I was inspecting my feet, and pushed it through the fence onto the ground.

If you're thinking, jeez, why couldn't she follow those clearly diagrammed steps on the back of the box for the use of the menstrual apparati? Well, then let me tell you about my friend Anne. She went around an entire day with a whole tampon, pink plastic applicator and all, inserted up herself. She came home from school and said, "No way am I wearing these, Ma. They hurt like hell."

With all these menstruation nightmares, why on earth did we ever call it our "friend"? In junior high, we'd say, "I can't go to practice today because I have my *friend.*" Or one of us would stand 10 feet in front of another girl, look over our shoulder and ask, "I have my *friend*, does it show?" Translation: I have a huge diaper-like wadola of cotton between my legs. Do you think the boys will notice it in these skintight jeans?

The worst menstrual nightmares of all may have been suffered not my me, but by my father and two brothers. There were six bleeding women — my four sisters, my mother and I — in my house during a peak couple of years after my pubescence but before I went to college. A strange thing tended to happen — our menstrual cycles would synchronize, loosing unto the household six raving, crying, acne-prone, budding feminists fighting over clothes, bathroom, telephone, bad breath, stupidness, and conceitedness. Anything. You name it, we fought about it.

My mother once threw a clock radio at my head. I'm sure this was in a menstrual fugue state because she was normally a sweet, brownie-baking, do-your-science-fair-project-the-night-before kind of mother. She completely denies this incident, by the way, but it is in my dairy of 1975, along with much other blackmail fodder.

I wish my father, my brothers, and every man could experience just one menstrual cycle. That reminds me of a joke I heard many years ago. A guy meets a woman in a bar and wants to take her back to his place. She says, "I can't, I have my menstrual cycle." He says, "That's okay. I'll follow you on my moped." Just a word of caution: Don't try this joke at a staff meeting.

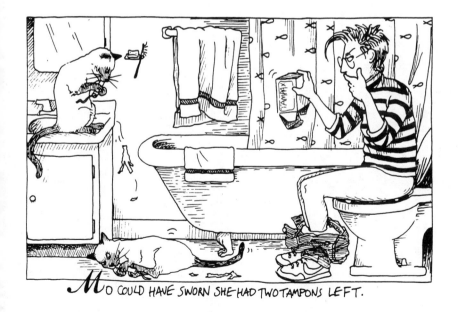

MO COULD HAVE SWORN SHE HAD TWO TAMPONS LEFT.

Cartoon by Alison Bechdel

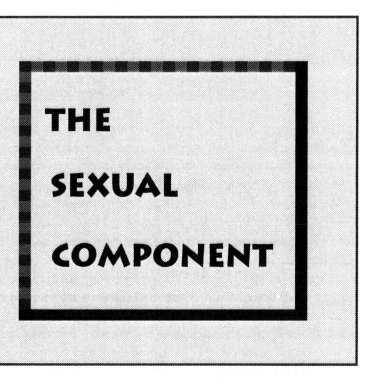

THE SEXUAL COMPONENT

What Is This Thing Called Libido?

by Cathy Crimmins

"Remember how you've been talking about your sex drive going up?" says my friend Louise over the phone. "I'm starting to feel the same way. All of a sudden I want to make love several times a day, preferably with different a man each time."

We joke nervously for a while and the conversation concludes with me officially welcoming her into the Horny Older Woman club. "God send us husbands, young and fresh a-bed!" I say, a salute taken from Chaucer's libidinous Wife of Bath.

Louise is 36 and I am 38. We are each long married and have four-year-old daughters. Since becoming what my husband affectionately calls "a sex maniac," I have been rather surveying my friends to see if my increased desire is normal or just some kind of premenopausal madness. So far, Louise is one of only a few who has satisfied my curiosity.

In my twenties and early thirties, I never thought much about my libido. I enjoyed making love, but sexual flashbacks and daydreams didn't occupy my spare time the way they do now. It seems that I was sleepwalking through the early years of my sexuality, including a disastrous first marriage that surely was motivated by sex, since we had little else in common.

But once I hit 35, I awakened with a start to discover that the whole world was about sex. How could I not have seen it before? I had spent my life being a smart girl, when what I really wanted to be was a sex kitten. I'm not complaining. This surge in libido has acted like a tonic, made me lighthearted and confident, and given new life to my marriage. Like the best things in life, it has come as a total surprise, and I'm still somewhat mystified as to its origins.

As a kid, all my sexual information came from the women's magazines my mother brought home from the supermarket. Once I found among the recipes and thinner thigh exercises an article detailing the sexual phases of a woman's life. When I got to the part where the doctor-author claimed that a woman in her late thirties can be preoccupied by sex as much as a 19-year-old boy, I felt sick to my stomach. Gross! Pathetic, I thought. That was my mother's age group then, and I couldn't imagine my mother even having sex, let alone thinking about it. But the signs of sexual preoccupation were there, I just didn't recognize them. My mother had developed a huge crush on Paul Newman and kept his poster on our refrigerator to torture my father, and she and her girlfriends were always sitting around in the kitchen discussing good-looking movie stars in a dreamy fashion.

My friends and I are a little less subtle when it comes to movie talk. "Boring missionary sex, but the guy does have a great butt," pronounced my friend Joellen when reviewing *The Lover*. "So-so movie, except for this incredible sex scene on top of a dirigible," I tell her in describing *Map of the Human Heart*. My attitude toward cinematic experience has changed completely since I crossed the threshold into a libidinous life. Once a film aficionada who would cheerfully endure six-hour grainy movies made in obscure countries, I now think that movies aren't worth seeing unless they contain good sex.

Are all my hobbies these days just sex substitutes? I don't trust myself anymore. Bodysurfing, always a favorite, seemed like good, clean fun in my twenties. But skimming along the crest of a wave this summer, I wondered if the sport's orgasmic qualities had attracted me. And how about my lifelong fascination with growing vegetables and flowers? Now I walk into my garden and see sex everywhere. I am nearly moved to tears over the plight of my female Kiwi vine, who has been growing more wanton each year as the male specimens we buy die before they are able to make her fruitful. This year, a little suitor has survived and seems to be doing his best to grow big enough to fertilize her.

I'm developing a new hobby, too, one almost too embarrassing to mention. I like looking at men, preferably young, good-looking ones. I lust after them in my heart. How did this start? For years I never even noticed what men looked like. Either I am going out of my mind, or I am finally learning how to have fun.

Let's go with the fun theory. There's at least a vague biological basis. At 33, I had a child. I've always ever wanted one child, and so, in a sense, I've fulfilled my biological destiny. Sex is never going to lead to anything except pure pleasure from now on. Sounds good to me.

Maybe this increased libido is nature's way of protecting me from Madison Avenue, a sort of self-esteem vaccination for getting older. Sure, my thighs and stomach are sagging and I'm developing wrinkles, but I feel sexy, the sexiest I've ever felt.

Only one thing keeps me from wholeheartedly embracing my new identity as a Horny Older Woman: It's the pathetic image we've always had throughout the ages. People laugh at the middle-aged Wife of Bath's sexual appetites and feel disgusted by Mrs. Robinson's seduction of young Benjamin in *The Graduate*.

A middle-aged professor once told me that she couldn't appreciate the portrayal of the mature lovers in Shakespeare's *Antony and Cleopatra* until she herself was the same age. When I first saw Anne Bancroft in *The Graduate*, I was 13 and thought she looked like a silly old lady. Twenty-five years later, Mrs. Robinson seems awfully attractive and just about my age. Why is it so terrible that she acts on her fantasies? *The Last Picture Show* came out when I was 16 and easily disgusted by the idea that a woman in her late thirties would go to bed with a teenager. Seeing it again, the many subplots about high school students seem boring compared to the scenes of the older woman/younger man affair.

In the Wife of Bath's tale, a knight is forced to marry an old hag who has saved his life by giving him the answer to the question, "What do women desire most?" Women desire mastery, advises the old woman. Although the knight has avoided execution, he feels sentenced to a life of sexual unhappiness, tied to an old hag he must service every night in bed. Taking pity on him, the hag says she can transform herself into a beautiful young maiden, but that he will then have to cope with other men coveting her. He cannot make up his mind, so he lets her decide what to do. To reward him for giving her mastery in the relationship, she becomes beautiful.

I prefer to interpret this story as a fairy tale about the compensations of age. I turn to it frequently as I search for clues to my newfound sexual euphoria. Like the hag in the tale, I have gained a certain amount of mastery in life. At 38, I feel happy, secure enough to fantasize about men I'll never have, and, best of all, finally able to unleash my inner beauty in bed.

❖

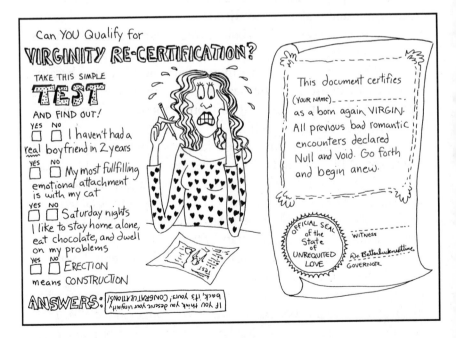

Cartoon by Libby Reid, from *Do You Hate Your Hips More Than Nuclear War?* (Penguin Books)

Raging Hormones

by Sheryl Wolff Kayne

Soon after my divorce, during a conversation about whether we had to make a trek to the grocery store in the middle of the day or if we could wait until evening, my 13-year-old daughter suddenly changed the subject. "Mom, I guess now that you are divorced, it must mean you're not getting any."

Hmmm. My first reaction was to say, "I hardly ever got any while I was married," but I figured that that was inappropriate, so I didn't. My second reaction was, "I hate to be the first one to tell you this, but sex is not only for teenagers." That wouldn't have been appropriate either, so I opted for a different tack.

"I am exactly where I want to be right now," I reassured her. "I am very happily unmarried and I am sure I will be meeting lots of nice people and making good friends."

I guess she was thinking about divorced parents' sexual patterns because her father had jumped into a series of hot-and-heavy relationships immediately after moving out, and I hadn't. I became a homebody, devoting my time and energy to my kids and my work, day in and day out, for the first six months following "The Big D." Then the raging hormones hit.

My lips kept wanting to pucker; my arms ached to hold someone. My spine and back muscles yearned to be rubbed, just that right wonderful way. I wanted to smell a guy up close and personal. My voice jumped two octaves every time I talked to a male. Sexy scenes on television brought tears to my eyes. I was in a very uncomfortable, constant state of yearning.

I knew what I wanted to do, but "Sexually Experienced" was not my middle name.

I got married at 19 to the only man I'd ever known, in the biblical sense. Being born again as a single woman in the '90s, I felt as though I'd been a freeze-dried pea, lost at the bottom of a huge deep freeze for a millenium, that was then popped into a microwave and emerged as a vegetable medley.

I got married on the sexual cusp — caught between the years when good girls didn't and everybody did. The sexual revolution marched right by me, with barely a climax. I spent 20 years in a chastity belt.

Although the lock was now broken, being married had definitely stunted my sexual growth. After a lifetime of relating to only one man, I wasn't exactly emotionally equipped to run out and go to bed with the first person I met. Not that there weren't opportunities.

I said no thanks to the long line of men who came to fix an assortment of things at my house — the married carpenter, the married lawn guy, the gorgeous, older, married roof guy. My motto became, "I don't do married men."

I considered running a personal advertisement: "Unmarried raging hormones needs to meet single male with like affliction. ASAP."

Instead, I did something I never thought I'd do. I went to a singles' discussion group that meets weekly. The first week's topic was, "Is it harder to find romance or friends?"

The following week's discussion on "Does she, or doesn't she? You never know when you're going to get it," was really up my alley. The more I talked and the more people I met, the better I felt.

My raging hormones toned down to a simmer.

I continue going to the meetings and being with people like me who are parents busy raising children and promoting careers who also recognize the need to have close friendships without long-term commitments. People to call for a hug, a movie, a backrub.

I often think about that conversation with my daughter. I spoke the truth. I am exactly where I want to be right now, happily un-married, meeting lots of very nice people, making good friends.

Anaïs Nin's To-Do List

by Andrea Carlisle

Monday
Sweep barge
Write in journal
Sleep with Henry
Sleep with June
Sleep with husband
Sleep!

Tuesday
Sleep with husband
Sleep with June
Sleep with Henry
Write erotica — eight pages
Seek dancing, friendships, nature,
forgetfulness, music, etc.

Wednesday
Sleep with June?
Sleep with Henry
Sleep with hubby
See man about erotica — collect $8
Diary (record *everything*)
Ponder the ego
Get some rest

Thursday

The Diary — don't hold back!
Sleep with H & J
Husband out of town — drop him a lusty note
Order:
50 new journals
2 gallons ink
20 good fountain pens
Erotica — 10 pages!
(Cape in window at Z's: $10)
Rediscover Spanish blood with G —
passion, fire, warmth, fervor, and so on
Work on novel (remember to write as *a woman*)
Try to get to bed early

Friday

Diary (whole hog)
Soak writing hand in Epsom salts bath
Collect $10
Buy cape, shoes, wide-brimmed hat
Sleep with Henry and June and husband
Ponder neurosis
Smoky bar
Erotica — 12 pages, nothing less will do
Beddy-bye

❖

Pill Stories

by Lisa Jansen

When a woman starts taking the Pill, she's told how important it is to take it at the same time every day. There are more rules to follow if you don't and scary consequences if you miss the time more than once a month. Those of us who have been on the Pill for a while have worked it into our daily routines, but we remember when taking it at the same time every day was a challenge. In my circle, we call these our "Pill Stories."

One roommate — I'll call her Sheryl — decided 6 a.m. was the best time to take her Pill. As a college student with an erratic schedule, it was the only time of day she could consistently count on being in the same place — in bed. Every morning at 6 a.m., the alarm would go off and Sheryl would stumble to the bathroom to take her Pill. At least, we assumed it was the Pill. Without her contacts she was legally (and obviously) blind, but every day she took something at 6 a.m. One morning, her boyfriend stumbled into the bathroom instead, and he took something. I guess it worked — they made it through med school and law school without getting pregnant.

Another roommate, Mary, would "forget" to take her Pill for days at a time. More than once, when she was having a tough time in school, she hinted that maybe she'd like to have a baby, instead. She shared this thought with her roommates but, of course, neglected to mention it to her boyfriend. The household went on a campaign to make sure Mary took her Pill on time. We never had to sneak it in with her hamburger or dissolve it in her orange juice, but we did have to quiz her every night around 7 p.m.

Lydia had it easier — most of the time. One year out of school and working full time, she had a pretty regular schedule. Her Pill time was noon. One day she stood at a drinking fountain, mouth filled with water, ready to take her Pill. She tipped her head back and popped the Pill, but somehow it missed her mouth and flew past her head. She dropped to the ground, frantically searching for the

Pill. An older man (a priest? her second grade piano teacher? the Republican Senator she hadn't voted for in November?) who had been walking by offered to help. Flustered, Lydia told him she had lost an earring back. The man picked up something, examined it, said, "Oh, it's just somebody's pill," and tossed it into a nearby stairwell.

Half an hour later, when the coast was clear, Lydia found her Pill on the stairs. ❖

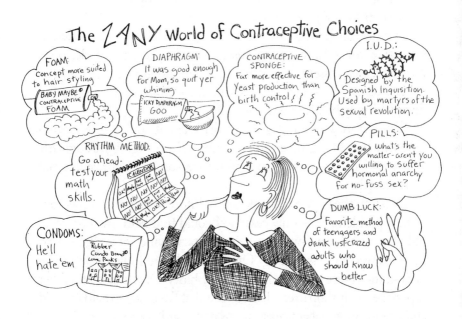

Cartoon by Libby Reid, from *Do You Hate Your Hips More Than Nuclear War?* (Penguin Books)

Sizzling

by Donna Ann Black

You've probably noticed all the "add spice to your sex life" magazine articles that appear all the time. One in particular caught my attention: It described a guaranteed way to make me and my lovemate "sizzle" in sexual anticipation.

You see, with two young children running around in circles (which keeps me and their dad running around in circles), there's not a whole lot of time for anything else, and after all that running, any free moments are usually spent resting.

But sizzling sounded like such a red-hot idea, I felt I had to give it a try. So I read the article's instructions and learned that, basically, all I had to do was get one tape recording of me and my lovemate fooling around. And if I could tape it without my partner's knowledge, so much the better, for that was supposed to add even more sparks at playback time.

Not usually keen on having anything I do be taped, I decided to put aside my misgivings because, according to the article, once recorded, this cassette would be an instant aphrodisiac guaranteed to take us to new heights of afternoon (or morning or nighttime) delight simply by playing it!

But before I could play it, I had to tape it, and before I could tape it, I had to dig up a tape recorder. Rummaging through my two-year-old's toy chest, I spotted my treasure: a bright yellow Big Bird recorder.

Next on the list was a blank tape. Unfortunately, this turned out to be a problem. The only cassette I could find held my four-year-old's tap recital song, but after a momentary twinge of guilt, I erased it. Sure, we'd all miss hearing "On the Good Ship Lollipop" but to be honest, the choice between listening to Shirley Temple sing about her trip to the candy shop to eat all the sweets that I'm trying so hard to avoid and sizzling in sexual anticipation was not a hard one to make.

Having procured the necessary "pre-sizzle" components, all that was left was the taping. As luck would have it, an opportunity to perform the final deed presented itself on Saturday morning. For as soon as the kids finished their usual breakfast of cereal, toast, and bananas dipped in picante sauce (they're both native Texans), two fat little bodies wobbled out of the kitchen and into the living room to watch cartoons.

So, as the girls sat entranced with Bugs Bunny, Donald Trump (I mean Duck), and all their animated buddies, I quickly awakened my nearly asleep spouse, and by mid-morning, both the tape recorder and newly-taped-on cassette were safely hidden under my side of the bed (the only place I knew the kids wouldn't go because that's where monsters live). And although I had been able to keep it a secret from my spouse, I must admit I was really tempted to immediately play it back for myself, but then I remembered that the article stressed that the listening should be a "together" experience.

Knowing that a long night of wining, dining, and being "together," wouldn't be possible with two young children close by, I called the grandparents. With just minimal begging and my signing on a notarized note promising I'd replace whatever got broken, they agreed to baby-sit at their house.

The big night arrived and after finishing a lovely meal made even more special because we didn't have to dodge catapulting, toddler-size silverware or spend hours removing bits of food from the walls, table, and chairs, we retired to the bedroom.

I lit some candles (actually a whole bunch — we only had the small birthday kind) and put on my sexiest T-shirt. Well, okay, it was the same T-shirt I wore every night, but at least I didn't accessorize it with my usual thermal ankle socks, and my face wasn't smeared with its usual glob of anti-aging wonder cream.

Winking seductively at my husband (he asked if I had something in my eye), I retrieved the tape recorder and cassette. While he jokingly asked if we were going to "tap off" our dinner (See, I told you we'd all miss the Good Ship Lollipop), I snuggled next to my lovemate, told him I had a grand surprise and hit the play button.

As it turned out, there was a heckuva surprise in store for both of us. I suppose we could have sizzled in sexual anticipation, but that's tough to do while you're doubled over laughing with tears streaming out of your eyes. You see, our aphrodisiac recording went something like this:

"Gee, Honey, guess it's been a while; do you remember how to do this?"

"No, I really don't but I read somewhere that you never forget how to ride a bike, so maybe if we got on top of your old 10-speed, this would come back as well."

"MMMmmm you smell really good — like strawberry jam — oh, wait a minute, you've got a big glob of it in your hair."

"Great. I was wondering where Annie left her piece of breakfast toast. Do you see any slightly burned bread nearby?"

"Oh no. Did you hear that?"

"Hear what? I found the bread, she stuck it in my ears."

"I think I just heard Brooke tell Annie she shouldn't have taken her diaper off because it was making the new couch wet."

"We'd better hurry and finish."

Knowing that laughter is the best medicine, I figure if we play the tape once a day, we'll never get sick. And when the offspring are finally grown and living elsewhere, we'll still be healthy enough to have our long, romantic interludes and who knows, maybe we'll even sizzle. ❖

SYLVIA   by Nicole Hollander

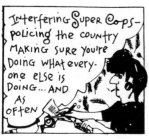 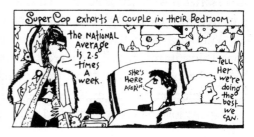

Cartoon by Nicole Hollander

Self-Service

by Nina Silver

There once was a woman named Doris
Who spent her time with her clitoris.
She expertly knew
All the right things to do,
Saying, "Anyone else would just bore us."

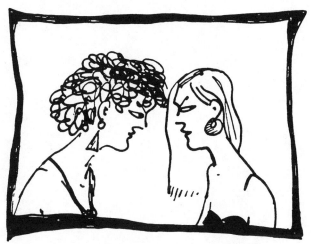

"I call it bore-play.
That's when he spends
3 hours touching you...
in the wrong place!"

Cartoon by Stephanie Piro from *Men! Ha!* (Laugh Lines Press)

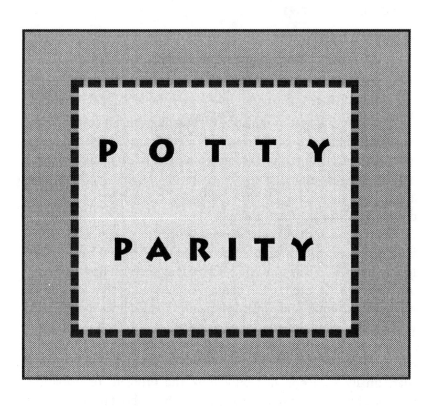

A Bladder Matter
by Nina Silver

The Moon Also Rises
by Dorothy M. Sheils

A Bladder Matter

by Nina Silver

Several years ago in the state of Washington, an enterprising college student set up camp in front of a public rest room with a box lunch, a digital counter, and a stopwatch. The lunch would come in handy, for she intended to be there all day. As each female approached the women's bathroom door, click went her meter. She did the same for the men's room.

At the end of the day, the student tallied her scores. The results should not surprise anyone: The average time women had to wait to use their toilets was triple that of how long the men had to wait to use theirs. As the result of this young woman's study, state legislation was passed to equip and expand women's toilet facilities so that their waiting time would be equivalent to men's.

We've all seen lines for women's bathrooms at movie theaters, concert halls, restaurants, and schools. It gives me great pleasure that, finally, someone not only took the problem of urination seriously, but had the initiative to do something about it. I fervently wish that all of America reconsider its toilet habits. There should be more toilets for women because of women's physiology.

One might think that in an enlightened culture such as ours bathroom architects might pay special attention to the distress of female bladders. But the sad truth is that in our society, elimination functions are taboo, disdained, and loathed. Whether that's because the organ of peeing is also the organ of sexual desire, is a matter of debate. One could also argue that people are embarrassed about sex because it's so closely related anatomically to eliminating. But whichever way it goes, one thing is certain: Not only are Americans hung up about sex, they are equally, if not more, in the dark about urination.

I have never been bathroom-secretive with any of my lovers or my close friends. These friends — who usually do not walk around nude — don't mind if the bathroom door is open when they're using the toilet. In fact, they prefer it open. How else can they continue talking to me without interrupting the flow of conversation when they need to get rid of a little extra water? And should I wait until one friend finishes putting on her makeup if I really need to be on the toilet? Why be so cruel to my body?

And what about the euphemisms we use for equipment or places designated for elimination of our waste material, the products of food combustion? You see signs all over for public rest rooms. Really. Do people rest in these rest rooms? And what about bath room? A bathroom or bath house contains precisely that, a bath or baths. Europe is famous for them. When our British cousins, for example, mean toilet, they say so. In America, hardly anyone today utters the word toilet. Why?

And what about those ludicrous universal symbols on the doors: an angular figure in pants and an equally crude figure in a dress? Never mind that some women never wear dresses, or that many don't wear them all the time. Perhaps when we're wearing pants, we should have access to the men's room? Not long ago, in a movie theater where there was the typical long line in the women's room, three other women and I resolutely marched to the "pants" facility and took it over. The man using the urinal looked surprised, but we courteously waited for him to leave before doing what we needed to do.

Until we can remedy the shortage of women's facilities (do we need an act of Congress? Come to think of it, Congress didn't even have a women's toilet until 1992), women should, in a gesture of self-love, commandeer the "pants" facility whenever the "dress" one is overpopulated. If you're a man, just get in line behind your smaller-bladdered sisters. And after you've finished, don't forget to put the seat down.

A bladder matter should be everyone's concern. Next time, the bladder on overload might be your own.

❖

The Moon Also Rises

by Dorothy M. Sheils

My daughter, Joan, and I had landed in Luxembourg, rented a car, and were on the road no more than five minutes when we spotted it. A dazed young couple in a van with a large homemade sign attached to the rear panel that proclaimed to the world, "WE ARE LOST IN EUROPE." Joan and I looked at each other smugly. "Ha," I said. "That'll never happen to us." Those were my last coherent words for the next three weeks.

One of those little unexpected surprises occurred while we were driving along the German autobahn on our way to the medieval town of Bacharach nestled along the Rhine River valley. We were on the outskirts of Stuttgart, breezing along at our usual 100 miles per hour, when we noticed that traffic was gradually slowing down. In no time at all four lanes of cars came to a dead stop. It was then that we realized that this was the last day of Oktoberfest and we were caught in the mass exodus of weary travelers from those fair grounds. But we were optimistic; the large sign on our right informed us that we were only 1,000 meters from our exit.

For the first two hours we read, played word games, conversed with other motorists, and enjoyed the ingenuity of the four young men in the convertible in front of us. Each time the traffic crawled a few more feet they'd all jump out and push their car forward. We all applauded their efforts, and they responded with deep bows of appreciation.

As we settled into the third hour of motionless irritation it suddenly became clear to me that the cold, foamy beers I had quaffed with relish at lunch were now seeking to emerge. I shifted uncomfortably. I wriggled. I bounced. My heels and toes tapped a wild beat to unheard music. Finally, in desperation, I got out of the car and walked a half mile or so scanning the horizon. To no avail: That stretch of the autobahn was as barren as the Sahara. On my way back I noticed that I wasn't alone in my predicament. Many faces held a pained expression, and lots of eyes rolled heavenward in silent supplication. It failed to console me, and the sight of little boys jumping out of cars to turn their backs on waiting traffic and let nature take its course filled me with envy.

Twilight and the fourth hour descended while my bladder bloomed and stretched to alarming proportions. I had visions of it being surgically removed. As we slipped into the fifth hour the traffic started to crawl and we finally made the exit, but so did every other car, all looking for the blessed sign that would read REST PLATZ. The area was jammed and we had to triple-park alongside a huge tandem truck. Joan raced to search for the rest rooms only to find that this was a picnic area with no facilities.

All the cars had turned off their lights and I became aware of how dark it was. As my eyes became accustomed to the darkness and the pale light of the full moon trickled through the leaves, I beheld a sight that is burned in my memory for all of eternity. For one split second my mind flashed back to a course I had taken in astronomy where I learned that the planet Jupiter had 10 to 12 moons, but the sight before me made that knowledge obsolete. For there before me, long lines of women were gratefully mooning the German countryside; privacy and modesty had fled in the wake of that five hour wait. With a cry of joy I ran forward and, clutching the rim of a trash barrel, I stooped to conquer, and added yet another moon over Stuttgart.

❖

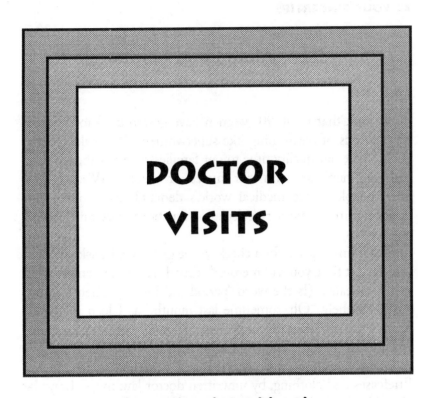

DOCTOR VISITS

Sometime Last Month
by Gyl Elliott

Taking Time for What's Important
by Sheryl Kayne

To Prep or Not To Prep
by Sheryl Kayne

Biological Options
by Cathy Crimmins

A Vagina of One's Own
by Inga Muscio

Take a Good Look
by Debra Gussman, M.D.

Sometime Last Month

by Gyl Elliott

I think that most '90s women have gotten used to the high expectations of performing like superwomen. We make the big bucks, mete out quality time to our families, take out the garbage, and communicate with our mates or dates. What I find unreasonable is the medical world's demand that women also perform complex memory/calculation functions every time we visit our doctors.

Each time I go in for a checkup, the gynecologist asks, "When was the last time you had menses?" First I have to remember what menses means. (Is the word "period" off limits?) Then I always answer blithely, "Oh, sometime last month," as I lean frantically toward my briefcase for an answer. I know that "sometime last month" isn't specific enough, but dressed in a backless gown and completely without reference material, it's the best I can do. Briefcases and clothing, by unwritten doctor law, must always be placed in the farthest corner of the examining room. My holy grail of information and security is hopelessly far away in a corner.

Making any desperate movement is dangerous while wearing the stunning white paper tearaway suit we've all grown to tolerate. I abandon my efforts to move when the paper suit becomes more stuck to the vinyl table than to me. Instead, I try to recollect the momentous occasion. These days, menses memories are not on the top of my list. Most of the time, I feel lucky if I get the date on my checks right.

"Now, exactly when?" she asks, still writing. (What are they always writing?) In desperation, I look around for clues.

Standard issue in every gynecologist's office is a tiny calendar, always on the wall farthest from the patient. My next attempt is to read this calendar, counting backwards from today to remember when, exactly, I tried to eat all the peanut butter from the jar and throw it at the dog at the same time. That would have been the beginning of my PMS phase.

After guessing at an appropriate date, she asks how long my menses lasted. Is this a trick question? I didn't know this kind of information would be on the test when I started, or I might have opted out altogether.

Another round of calculations (how many days did I wear pants that week?) and I come up with another guess. After absorbing this precious information, the doctor proceeds to reward my efforts with an internal exam. This is always the time when I wonder if we really need to visit a gynecologist twice a year, or if it's all a hoax concocted to provide the medical profession with expensive sports cars.

Are men required to remember things like this? If so, exactly what things would they be? And should we be writing things like this in our business calendars along with "fiscal year budget meeting at three"? Maybe menses notes should be added to the other information tables lumped in the back of those expensive calendar books. It could be in there even now, but who has time to go through all that "key information" and "ready reference" stuff?

This is just another example of the "second shift" at work. Women not only have to work longer for less pay, we also have to remember monthly bodily functions and recite them from memory on demand. If you take into account the potential number of brain cells lost in bearing children (my sister with two children insists that this is a fact), then storing this information along with everything else puts many women dangerously close to memory overload. We could crash our hard drives trying to keep track of menses.

After much musing on this memory dilemma, I have come up with a modern, '90s solution. Every month on menses day, the patient calls the doctor's office automated number. After "Press 11 to hear this message in Farsi," there will be a message saying, "If today is your first day of menses, please input your medical account number after the beep." Now, what's my medical account number?

Taking Time for What's Important

by Sheryl Kayne

Just yesterday, when my mother wanted me to take the afternoon off from work to take her shopping, I said no. I felt terrible about it, but I just couldn't afford the time.

I like my mother and I like shopping, but I had so much work to do, I didn't even eat lunch. I worked straight through. Sometimes I'm so busy, I literally do not take time to go to the bathroom.

Last night, my youngest daughter was in a cello concert, followed by my oldest playing her saxophone with the school band, after which she sang with a barbershop quartet in a coffee house 45 minutes away from our home. Of course, I drove her both ways and came home in between to throw dinner together, but I didn't even have time to read the newspaper. I hate that feeling of not having an extra moment for anything.

But I've learned my lesson. After days, weeks, months, and years of surviving on a schedule more appropriately kept on a roller coaster wheel than a wall calendar, I finally threw my hands up in the air and said, "Hey, Sheryl, this is your life."

When the children are grown, my work is done, and the garden is weeded, no one is going to turn to me and say, "Sorry you didn't have time to do the really important things in life."

No. No one will care but me. So I'm standing up for my rights. From now on, I am going to make time for what's really important. I will prioritize and organize my life properly. I will make the time for a yeast infection.

When that itchy feeling starts, I will stop what I am doing and enjoy the moment. At that first discharge of fluids, I will respond in a positive way, "This is a yeast infection. I have time for it."

As I plug in my heat lamp with my right hand, I will cancel my day's appointments with my left. I know today will give me those special moments I need alone, in private, just me and my yeast infection.

I remember my very first one. It seemed so mild, so mellow, a simple little itch that did not properly forewarn me of what could be coming my way.

It came before the days of Mycelex 7 and Gyne-Lotrimin over the counter. I had to call my gynecologist to report, "I have a yeast infection."

"How do you know?" he asked.

"I have a vaginal discharge resembling freshly made cottage cheese. My vagina feels like it is on fire and my fingernails are firmly entrenched between my legs to attack this itch from hell."

"Is the discharge odorous or green in color?"

"No, it is slightly off-white and rather pleasant smelling."

"I'll call in a prescription for vaginal inserts to be used for seven days. In the meantime, refrain from sexual intercourse, do not use soap on your lower body, only wear cotton panties, and no panty-hose."

"Will that make it go away forever?"

"Works for me." He lied.

One year — to the day — later, that familiar itch from super hell returned. At least it had waited long enough for the Food and Drug Administration to put the remedies on the pharmacy shelf. I went shopping to pick my own cure.

Oh, there's Mycelex 7, Summer's Eve and Gyne-Lotrimin, clotrimazole vaginal suppositories, 100% natural, hypoallergenic, sodium-free, noncaloric douche, and vaginal antifungal creams, to name just a few. The over-the-counter remedies in my local grocery store numbered 17 varieties. And I only have one vagina.

I tried Monistat-7 because of their enclosed educational pamphlet and warning: "Do not take by mouth." I felt that was truly responsible advertising, packaging, and consumer protection, all in one. I was cured, until the following month when that all too familiar itch returned, which made me realize it was time to further investigate my problem.

The commercial products can make the symptoms of vaginal infections disappear; however, if the infections reoccur, there's a reason. In my case, continual use of antibiotics for chronic sinus infections led me down that cruel, painful, vaginal yeast infection path. My solution was vitamin therapy, incorporating Primado-philus, a lactobacillus and acidophilus capsule, into my daily regimen. I needed to replace the good bacteria in my system, which were being killed off by the constant use of antibiotics.

Yes, thanks, I'm doing much better. Most importantly, I've reminded myself how very important I am. My health and daily needs are just as significant as everyone else's.

I will no longer be one of those women so tied up with her children, work, house, home, beautiful garden, grocery store chores, dry cleaning, dance, music, singing, art and pottery lessons to ignore the nitty-gritty side of my life that reminds me who and what I am.

My fellow sisters, I recommend that you do the same and you, too, will feel the benefits. When that next yeast infection calls, don't be too busy to answer. Make time for it and you will truly be a better person for it all.

The Cure

"Every woman has probably had at least one yeast infection, however, many others suffer from them repeatedly," says Pearlyn Goodman-Herrick, naturopathic physician from Weston, Connecticut. "They are most commonly caused by too much sugar in the diet, antibiotics destroying the good lactobacilus bacteria, which keep yeast in check, birth-control pills, and/or stress.

"The basic remedies that help include cutting out sugar from the diet, increasing B vitamins, and eating yogurt with acidophilus or a live culture."

Dr. Goodman-Herrick also suggests a vinegar douche to relieve discomfort, once a day for three consecutive days: Mix two tablespoons of apple cider vinegar in one pint of warm water. The apple cider vinegar helps kill off the yeast.

Follow the three days of vinegar douches with one day of a yogurt douche: two tablespoons of live-culture yogurt with one pint of water. Then repeat the four-day cycle.

Other remedies include douching with yarrow or grapefruit seed oil extract. Some women find relief for acute yeast infections by inserting a clove of peeled garlic into the vagina. Dr. Goodman-Herrick says the clove should be changed on a daily basis and will stay in place like a tampon. The major drawback is that in the morning, the garlic user will wake up smelling from garlic oils carried into the bloodstream.

"There are two points of view in treating yeast infections," says Dr. Goodman-Herrick. "One is the over-the-counter approach. When the symptoms disappear, the problem is cured. But if vaginal infections reoccur, there's a problem with the underlying system. Classic homeopathy, for example, treats each woman constitutionally to strengthen her overall system. I do not see a yeast infection as separate from what goes on with the rest of the person. It is very important to look at each person as a totality."

To Prep or Not To Prep

by Sheryl Wolff Kayne

Election day, November 2, 1976. Two weeks before my due date with my first child. It was also the day I was scheduled to sit for my graduate board exams in school psychology. I'd spent the entire summer and fall months preparing for this three-hour exam with the reputation that only one third of the people taking it would pass.

I was tense. I was anxious. I was a basket case.

My neighbor Dave called first thing in the morning and offered to drive me to the local voting booth in his royal blue, four-in-the-floor Datsun. We laughed and joked while the low sports car took every bump and pothole in the road. I voted. Returned home. Went to the bathroom and saw puddles of blood.

I decided against an overall panic. I simply became mildly hysterical as I phoned my obstetrician. For the first time in nine months, my phone call was put directly through. However, my usual doctor was off. His partner was on.

Even though I knew the office rules when I joined the practice, "alternate doctors with each visit so that you will get to know them both," I hadn't. I went with this practice because I knew that both doctors did Lamaze deliveries.

But it was Dr. Appleberg who had been recommended to me. He was funny and sensitive to my needs. I liked him and felt comfortable with him. Even though I knew these two doctors covered each other for deliveries, I had only met Dr. Morris once.

I didn't like him very much. He was a much older man, who spoke with a very thick, European accent I found difficult to understand. As many wonderful things as I'd heard about Dr. Appleberg, Dr. Morris had received mixed reviews.

I remember anxiously staring at the clock, counting the hours until my exam, feeling the dark, scary warmth of my stains, listening to Dr. Morris dictate to me what had to be done, immediately.

"Get in bed and stay there. Since you are not feeling any other symptoms or pain, an internal exam might stir up more problems.

72

Remain in bed for the next 24 hours and keep in close touch with the office."

"I have to take a three-hour exam this afternoon for my master's degree. If I don't take it today, I have to wait until May when it's offered again. I've been studying around the clock."

"Change your sanitary pad now so you can judge if there's any increase in the staining or if it's minimal. As long as it doesn't increase or it stops, I'd say go ahead and get the exam out of your way. The tension alone could cause the staining. Good luck."

Wow. He sounded so civilized. So caring. So sensible. Maybe what I'd heard about him wasn't really true. Deep down, I knew not to open up a can of worms right before the exam, but I had to ask. I had to know the truth. "I've heard you require a special kind of prepping before delivery. What does that mean?"

"Perhaps you are referring to my instructions that nurses are to shave the patient's pubic area in preparation for delivery?"

"It's true! I've never heard of that before. Why do you do that?"

"It used to be very common. I find that women are very unclean, dirty even, and it is healthier and more efficient to cleanse the area completely by removing the hair."

I started defending myself and my pubic hair. "I'm not very hairy at all. My hair is sparse and short and smooth and has never gotten in the way before. You can actually see my skin through the pubic hair, it's that thin and sparse. And I'm very clean. And how can you say something like that, that women aren't clean?"

With each sentence I uttered, I felt another stain spurt out. For once in my life, I lacked the energy to fight, yet I was so furious I had trouble speaking.

The thought of shaving off my pubic hair horrified me. At that point in my life, I didn't even shave my legs. The thought of a tiny little stubble growing between my legs, rubbing against my thighs until it grew back in properly, enraged me.

"Okay, completely clean yourself at home," he quickly backed off. "I'll mark your chart that you don't have to be fully prepped."

I hung up the phone in a state of shock. I kept repeating to myself, "I can't deal with this now. Exam first, baby later. Exam first."

I stayed in bed for the afternoon, surrounded by research on psychological testing statistics and standards. The staining subsided. I showed up for the exam promptly at 5 p.m., was assigned a room, a proctor, a table, and table mate. At 5:20, I felt my first contraction.

I stared at the clock for the next 10 seconds and returned to the exam. At 5:40, my body shook with another round of contractions. My table mate called over the proctor, "Could you seat me somewhere else? I think she's in labor."

"Must be false labor," I cheerily replied, determined not to be back in this same room again in May. I was left alone to inhale sharply and chart my contractions every 20 minutes until I completed the exam.

I arrived home, totally exhausted. The contractions had stopped. The staining had stopped. I went to bed, knowing I'd need even more strength in the morning.

Eight a.m., I called Dr. Appleberg. "Will you guarantee me that you will deliver my baby?"

"It's a fifty-fifty chance you'll get me or Dr. Morris. You've known that from the beginning."

"I didn't know about the prepping then."

"I don't do that and he has waived you. It's on your chart."

"I can't support a doctor whose entire practice services women when he has such a poor view and total lack of respect for women."

Deep down, I knew I was over a barrel. The doctors' fees had been submitted to my insurance carrier at the beginning of the pregnancy and covered all costs through delivery and postnatal care.

I spent the morning calling obstetric/gynecological practices. Each conversation was the same, "For insurance purposes, we cannot begin with a new patient in the ninth month."

Decision time. I called the doctors' office back. "I'm due to deliver anywhere between November 12th and 15th. What is Dr. Morris's schedule?"

"He's on call November 11, 12, and 13," responded the receptionist, "and out of town November 14, 15, and 16."

I called my parents to tell them I'd be giving birth between November 14th and 16th. I instructed my husband that I would be spending November 11th through 13th in bed, resting, waiting for the 14th to deliver the baby.

Then I wrote a statement that Dr. Morris was not to deliver my child under any circumstances. I recognized that I was taking a chance, depending upon the availability of emergency backup services at the hospital, but I couldn't live with the notion of this man delivering my baby. I had it notarized and added to my medical chart.

At 12:01 A.M. on November 16, I went into labor. Elanit Dvora Kayne was born at 4:53 a.m., with Dr. Appleberg in attendance. At 5:30 a.m., I released both Drs. Appleberg and Morris as my physicians.

The telephone rang at 9:00 a.m. "This is Dr. Morris calling to inform you that I will no longer be requiring full preps of my patients."

"Good decision, but I still don't want to be affiliated with physicians who lack basic respect for their patients."

In my opinion, Dr. Morris had a barbaric view toward women. I should have known that before I chose his practice. With baby number two, I asked many more questions before selecting a doctor.

Above and beyond competent medical care, I sought a positive, caring attitude towards people, all people. Giving birth was the most magnificent experience of my life, twice.

To me, birthing and the people doing the birthing are beautiful. Absolutely beautiful. The people we decide to share this wonderful event with should be worthy of the honor and privilege.

❖

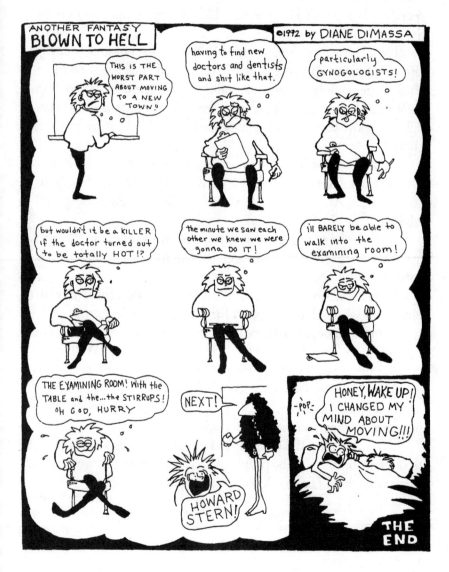

Cartoon by Diane DiMassa from *What Is This Thing Called Sex?* (The Crossing Press)

Biological Options

by Cathy Crimmins

I always expected to give birth in a hospital (preferably in a drug-induced stupor), but I didn't count on having personality conflicts with hospital staff. Actually, I wouldn't call them personality conflicts. More like personality nuclear wars.

I'm not a nice girl. I yell a lot when I get angry. Having to wait for hours on end in reception areas makes me angry. At my third prenatal appointment at the hospital, after about an hour cooling it on the delightful vinyl sofa, I began screaming and didn't stop until I got dragged into the inner office, where someone clapped a blood pressure cuff on me.

"You're going to be one of our high-risk patients," said the doctor, coming in and looking at the chart. "Your blood pressure is sky high."

"You're going to be at very low risk of ever seeing me again," I said, and left immediately (I never did return that hospital gown, either).

In the Yellow Pages under "Midwives" I found a listing for a "Little Birthing Center on the Prairie" type of place that was hyper-politically correct and never kept people waiting for more than five minutes, probably because they only had about 12 demented ex-hippie clients. A groovy quilt of a uterus and fallopian tubes hung on the wall, and the stirrups on the examination table were covered with gingham potholders. Everyone referred to my "partner" and didn't make any assumptions that the guy coming with me to childbirth classes had sired my kid. I liked this attitude because it meant I could always deny Al's paternity at any time during the labor process and feel comfortable.

This little brick farmhouse setup didn't have doctors or even a lot of bureaucratic red tape, but there was some paperwork involved in giving birth there. For weeks the midwife hounded us to submit our "birth plan," a detailed document about exactly how we wanted our birthing experience to proceed.

There were so many elements I wanted to include as part of the optimal birth experience (like starting off with Mel Gibson at the conception). But it became a burden to decide between so many options. Delivering our baby at a birth center started to seem too much like buying a car or choosing bathroom fixtures.

The sperm donor and I spent hours debating the pros and cons of different birthing strategies. Should I sign up for Jacuzzi labor? After all, Flipper was born under water. So maybe our kid would have his own sitcom someday. But how could I enjoy sitting in a Jacuzzi for 10 hours without a glass of white wine?

Then there was the option of giving birth standing up. This sounded good, because I wanted to look my thinnest as I was delivering. But a friend of mine had said that when her breathing exercises failed her, she spent most of labor hitting her husband really hard during each contraction. I thought I'd have a difficult time getting the right leverage to slug Al if I was standing up.

The birth center also wanted to know how many people were planning to attend, what our video needs would be, and whether we required space in the refrigerator for casseroles. This threw me for a loop, since the experience was starting to sound more like a catered bar mitzvah than a natural physical event. I didn't really want anyone at the birth; frankly, I wished that I didn't have to be there, either. And I certainly didn't want pictures taken until after our child had left my body.

So far, developing the plan seemed odd. But then, on one of the last visits the midwife hit us with the weirdest non-option of all. "I'm obliged to let you know that you will be disposing of your own placenta," she said, producing a document for us to sign.

Alan and I looked at each other in panic. She then explained that hospitals sell their old placentas to special placenta-retrieval services, but that the birth center didn't have enough to sell each month. So it was the clients' responsibility to dispose of it as they saw fit. Some people buried it under a tree, for example, she said.

"I think you should drive out of there and stash it in the nearest dumpster at some fast-food restaurant," said my friend Sandy when I told her about it.

Before this, Al and I had never really thought about the placenta at all. But knowing that it was coming home with us, we started to imbue it with a personality. We began seeing it as an evil twin of the baby we were about to have, and sifted through our list of rejected baby names to see what we would call it. We gave it Alan's last name, since we had decided that our daughter would have mine.

In the end, some of the options we picked worked out pretty well. I did try Jacuzzi labor and liked it, even though they made me leave the tub to actually give birth. Getting me out of hot water must have been difficult, since apparently I was thrashing around and yelling at Al, "Pull me out of this Jacuzzi and you're a dead man."

My mother contributed to the birthing experience by baking a nice casserole, and even decided to be in the room as K was born. Leaving to go home the next day, proudly clutching our new bundle of joy, we were taken aback as the nurse handed us what felt like a pound and a half of chopped meat wrapped in brown butcher's paper.

Yep, it was Placenta, whom we had forgotten all about in the excitement of our daughter's birth. And now it was ours forever, or at least until we decided what to do with it. At least we didn't need a separate car seat or snowsuit for it. We weren't living at home at the time (my remodeling illness had forced us to move temporarily to another apartment), so it would be impossible to bury Placenta in the backyard. And I had grown too attached to it to go the fast-food disposal route. So the only thing we could figure out to do was to take it home and freeze it.

I recommend this course of action, in case you ever have a placenta disposal problem. It gave Al something to do when people came to see the new baby — he could take the guys into the kitchen and show them the placenta in the freezer next to the Häagen-Dazs. The only problem was, when it came to actually burying the thing when we got back to our own house, we didn't know the proper procedure. Should we defrost it first in the microwave, or bury it still frozen?

We decided on the latter, and Al buried Placenta under a hydrangea bush about two months after our kid's birth. It was a simple ceremony. ❖

A Vagina of One's Own

by Inga Muscio

Ahhhh, Springtime.

Sunshine, flowers, birds, bees, unwanted pregnancies.

I once published an article about herbal abortion, and people from all over North America called and wrote to me after the fact, asking, in no uncertain terms, how they might herbally abort with a nice, steamy cup o' Baby Away Tea.

However, I couldn't publish a recipe for Baby Away Tea.

Mainly because I believe it takes a lot of corporate and media conditioning to convince people they have no control over their bodies. Years and years, in fact. Likewise, it takes a lot to convince people they have all the power imaginable and more, over their bodies and lives. Nobody's gonna be adequately conditioned by reading one article by one fool writer.

Still, I'd like to make an attempt to set the stage.

First of all, herbal abortion is not "the answer." It's true, self-induced abortion is much more empowering than throwing up one's hands, spreading one's legs, and planting one's feet in them stirrups as a complete stranger, however supportive she may be, coaxes out the life inadvertently planted in the womb with a suction device designed by some long forgotten dude.

The fundamental principle that needs to be addressed is knowing, understanding, and accepting your body, on your terms. It is an irrefutable fact that my body is mine, mine, all mine. Everything on my body, every limb and characteristic is my commodity, my blessing, my curse, my responsibility.

Since muscles, teeth and skin are relatively self-explanatory, I focus on parts of my body that befuddled me and got me into exam rooms in the past. Namely my reproductive expanse.

I decided this was a good place to begin exerting my power as a living being on this planet. Coming to such an irrefutable conclusion is, I believe, the first step in conditioning yourself on your terms.

For some, it may be hard to believe your body is your own. If you've been sexually abused, especially as a child, it may be hard to deeply and all-knowingly believe your body belongs to you and no one else. Nevertheless, I stand by my scientific conclusion. In order to claim your own stake of power, you must believe the bod you call home is your ball o' wax.

All rightie, agenda item numero uno. In order to know your body, a certain amount of investment must be made. We have been anti-taught about taking care of ourselves, paying attention to our bodies for signs, symptoms and conditions. This creates a climate where power is generated into dollar signs, amassed by large corporations, dedicated to "caring" for our bodies in our stead. Learning to be responsible for your body will take time, as learning to be unresponsible has. Be patient with yourself, your ignorance and your curiosity.

Now, high in the sky resides a uterine compass and it is called the moon. After you decide your body is your finely tuned hot rod to tool you around this earth as you desire, start noticing the moon. Buy yourself a lunar calendar. Put it where you'll see it every morning. Slap it up by the coffee maker, the bathroom mirror or above your bed. Wherever, just look at it every day. Notice where the moon is on the calendar. As often as possible, notice the moon in the sky. That's all you have to do, nothing fancy, just notice the moon. The clincher here is *consistency*. Watch the moon grow and recede every month. Be able to eventually wake up in the morning and know where the moon will be that evening without looking.

This is aligning yourself with the moon, a good idea since the moon has been teaching ladies about their insides since we developed eyeballs able to see that high.

When you get your period, make a (red) mark on your moon calendar. What did the moon look like when you got your period? What did it look like last month? Sooner or later, you'll get a rhythm going with the moon. You'll have your period every New Moon, every Waxing Moon or maybe you will get your period on the Full Moon one month, the next month on the Waning Moon, next on the New Moon and next on the Waxing Moon. It varies just fantastically. There is no way of knowing what your cycle is until you lunarly track it. Even then, it is likely to traverse throughout the year, but if you keep a good record and watch what goes on between your pussy and the moon, you'll be able to predict, *to the day*, when you start your period, *even if you are "irregular."* Again, like I say, this takes time. You may not have a full grasp on your cycle for six months or even longer.

Patience is a virtue.

As you begin to groove with your fine snatch and the moon, you'll be able to perform all kinds of neato-o miracles. You can figure when you're ovulating or if you're in for a hellish period. Nasties like yeast infections can be easily nipped in the bud because you'll be so *utterly hip* with yourself. All those faintly clairvoyant premenstrual dreams will take on a more lucid clarity and depth. Sex becomes more intense and ecstatic. Menstrual cramps diminish. Let's see, what else. Oh, yes, you can even start to determine when you will and won't get in the family way, if you investigate the matter fully.

O.K. You got the moon bit.

Now, your body releases an egg once a month. This egg sits around in your uterus, waiting for some sperm to show up. It is not stupid. After 12-24 hours, it figures no sperm's gonna take it on a hot date and it goes away. Sperm can live in your body anywhere from 72 hours to five days. What this is means is, if you get some sperm in your uterus up to one working week before your body releases its egg, you can get pregnant. When an egg is present, you are ovulating. Normally, not always, but normally, a woman ovulates half way through her menstrual cycle. Therefore, if you had your period when the moon was New, then there's a good chance you'll ovulate when the moon is Full.

One way to tell you are ovulating is by sticking your finger (middle finger's best) up your vagina and swiping it around your cervix. (This is the thing inside your pussy that feels kind of like a nose.) What you will find if you are ovulating, is snot. It's quite unmistakable. It doesn't have any odor or color, it's just snot. What it's there for is it creates a hospitable, cushiony vehicle for sperm to travel to your egg. The unique characteristics of ovulation snot are influenced by a rise of the hormone estrogen. Right after you ovulate, if you stick your finger up your vagina, you'll find this sticky, tacky, maybe curdy, white stuff. If the sticky white stuff is there, but no snot, figure you just ovulated. Estrogen decreases at the approach of your period and progesterone rises, making your vag dry up a tad. Before you ovulate, the discharge is more milky and creamy. As you get used to checking your pussy stuff, you'll be able to recognize what's what.

Another indication that you're ovulating is a slight twinge of pain in your lower abdomen. It doesn't feel like a menstrual cramp, it's more of a tight pinched nerve-type pain. If you masturbate, you can feel it after you come.

Also, I should probably add, when you are ovulating, you will often become insanely horny. You may feel the urge to couple with the kitchen table leg when you're ovulating, though I wouldn't necessarily take this as an ovulatory symptom.

Have you ever seen your cervix? You won't be disappointed. It really is a lovely thing and quite the venerable axis. Go to your local women's health center and ask for a small, medium or large plastic speculum (or see page 110 below to order *Personal Insights: A Self-Examination Kit for Women* designed by Dr. Debra Gussman). Along with the speculum, get an instruction sheet. Read it and ask any questions you may have before leaving. With your speculum, you can further investigate and learn of the wondrous vagina. What you will need, beside the speculum is a flashlight, possibly some lube, and a hand held mirror. Practice opening and closing the spec a few times before inserting. If you're completely unfamiliar with this apparatus, remember to ask the nice health clinic lady to show you how to work it. Keep in mind speculums are not designed for self-exams. It can be frustrating trying to get that thing to work right the first one or nine times, but try to relax. Tight muscles won't facilitate this maneuver.

To insert a speculum: lie down with some pillows under the small of your back. Spread them legs. Hold your pussy lips apart with two fingers of one hand. Insert the speculum sideways, longest handle facing your body. If things are parched down there, employ the lube, but use it sparingly because one of the main objectives here is to be able to see your juices in their natural element. Ya' won't be able to tell the lube from the juice if you lay it on too thick. Once you get the speculum in about halfway, turn it so it lays flat. You don't want to try to open it up when it's sideways. Gently insert it on in to the hilt and open it up. Whee! There's a little lock mechanism on these things, click it into place when you get it opened as wide as you can.

Mind, this is not the most comfortable feeling in the world, but it shouldn't hurt at all (unless you have an infection or open sores or something), so long as you don't pinch any o' that tender skin as you open the speculum. However, if you're not used to having things in your vagina, especially hard things, you may experience more discomfort at first. Keep trying. Remember to relax. Once the speculum is in, opened and locked, grab that flashlight and mirror. If you can't see your cervix, either you have a long vaginal canal or a shy cervix. For the latter, bear down like you do when taking a shit. That cervix will overcome its stage fright in a matter of seconds. If lots of flesh is bulging around the speculum, you probably need a larger size.

Take a good long perusal. Note the shape, color and texture of your cervix. It changes appearance according to where you're at in your cycle. If you're ovulating, you may see mucous, your cervix will be pulled higher up, it may be softer and larger than usual and the opening of your cervix, called the os, may be open slightly.

If your cervix looks kinda bluish or is indeed bright blue, you're quite likely preggers. Either celebrate or get ready for a hearty counseling session with your health care provider, whichever you're in a mind for.

One final word.

I've bitched about the Pill in the past, but there's no time like the present when it comes to bitching about the Pill. It makes a lady gain weight, diminishes sexual desire, keeps one's body in a state of mock pregnancy, obstructs the natural cycle and menstrual flow, causes heart problems, irritability, migraines, has been linked to breast cancer and chemically dictates one's entire physical agenda. If you are on the Pill, think of it like this: Your life and body are in the hands of the scientists at the Ortho-Novum factory.

Marcy Bloom, the director of Aradia Women's Health Center in Seattle, paints a different picture and I thought I'd throw it in for good measure. Says Ms. Bloom, "Whatever you say about the Pill is true; however, it is the most successful method of birth control as well, that's the Catch-22. For some women, the Pill is the only method that works, or the only one they're willing to use because either they don't want to touch their bodies, or their lover is very resistant to using condoms. Sometimes the Pill's the only psycho-social method a woman is willing to use, because all other methods require a woman to touch herself."

Sad, but true.

It is downright contradictory to get to know your body when the Pill is in charge of it. Even if you get off the Pill, it may take a year for your body to forgive you and start acting like a normal human being again. I have nothing nice to say about the Pill. It fucks you up. It was designed by men in white coats who sit in laboratories all day long. (Now, now, I know there are plenty of female white coat wearers out there, but they are scientists in a world where men have defined science.) These people have no business telling ladies how to fuck and what to do to keep from getting pregnant.

Science, as it is in this day and age, is not compatible with the female cycle. Science is irrational, sterile and ignorant. A woman's cycle is rational, magic, and eternally, intelligently intuitive. If you are gonna put your body in the hands of science, your body and your cycle will one day get you back for it, I can promise you that.

Find some other form of birth control, dammit.

Learning how your body functions is not just a good idea. It's your god-given right, and everyone should take full advantage of it. By relegating this right to various commercial and corporate fuckheads, who have no interest in you as a living being, much less as a woman, you are relinquishing your power to unworthy institutions.

The entire feminine hygiene section in stores is, in actuality, a battlefield. Every item sitting on those shelves is dedicated to keeping women and their bodies divided, therefore conquered.

There's an awsome amount of power jes' sitting there, right between your legs. Tap into it.

Peace.

Take A Good Look at Yourself

by Debra Gussman, M.D.

My interest in female genital self-examination dates from my own adolescent curiosity about my body. I remember struggling with a gooseneck lamp (which got very hot) and a mirror, with my feet on my desk, hoping that my siblings wouldn't walk in on me.

Later, as an OB/GYN resident at the Hospital of the University of Pennsylvania I had a patient who affected me deeply. She was a young mother of three who came in to discuss contraception and have a pap smear. She had a large, dark, irregular mole on her labia, which she agreed to allow me to remove, mostly because it was ugly. She wasn't certain how long it had been there, nor whether or not it had changed. It turned out to be a melanoma. Despite surgery and chemotherapy, my patient died of metastatic melanoma. How different things might have been if she had been more familiar with her own body.

Women are ready today to take a more active role in their own health care. Many women routinely do a breast self-examination. This widely accepted behavior may lead to much earlier detection of breast cancers. Additionally, there are many products available to allow people to evaluate their own health. There are home pregnancy tests, kits to identify the time of ovulation, kits to check the stool for blood not visible to the eye, urine test tapes and finger blood sticks to check for diabetes, blood-pressure monitors available in many supermarkets, a number of dental self-care products to prevent tooth and gum disease, and disposable otoscopes to evaluate children's ears for infection.

It is time to extend this attitude of care and self-examination to the female sexual organs. This part of the body has often received little attention from a self-help point of view because of embarrassment, ignorance, and cultural taboos. Unlike the face, which is easily seen in the mirror, or the breasts, which are readily available for self-examination, the genitalia are difficult to see with the typical household mirror and light.

The benefits of genital self-examination include:

- Learning to recognize what is normal and to observe changes;
- Seeking early evaluation of neoplastic and infectious diseases at an easily curable stage;
- Learning the cyclic changes of the vagina and cervix; to improve natural family-planning techniques or to optimize pregnancy achievement;
- Improved communication with health care providers.

I have found that during a gynecological examination I can decrease the patient's anxiety and increase her comfort level by using a mirror that allows a woman to see herself. Over the years, using a mirror and giving a "guided tour" of the patient's anatomy has become a routine part of the care I provide. Patients are very receptive to learning more about their bodies and becoming active participants in their health care.

I designed *Personal Insights: A Self-Examination Kit for Women* for my patients. One of the difficulties in female self-examination is the awkwardness of holding the light with one hand, the mirror with the other hand, and needing a third hand to move the flesh around to see the various structures. The kit contains a specially designed mirror that clips onto a light source. This design allows the woman to have the light and mirror in one hand, leaving the other hand free. *Personal Insights* also contains a narrow, smooth plastic speculum to allow women to see their vaginal walls and cervix. A lubricant is included to allow a comfortable insertion of the speculum. There are clear, easy instructions to teach women the correct name and appearance of the female structures and how best to see them.

As my patients have become more comfortable with genital self examination, an unexpected benefit has been realized. Women who can describe symptoms and signs to me accurately on the phone do not necessarily need to come in. For example, if a woman can describe a lesion on the labia, such as folliculitis or a boil, we can make a treatment plan over the phone. If the measures don't work, the woman will then come in for evaluation. However, if the measures do work, the cost and inconvenience of an office visit are avoided. Patients may also describe something that requires immediate attention and unnecessary delays are prevented.

In this age where capitated health care is becoming a reality, patients will need to be more responsible for their own care. Skill at genital self-examination will allow better communication between a woman and her health care provider.

Knowledge is power. The more we women know about our bodies the more control we will have. We can learn what is normal. We can use this knowledge to improve our health.

❖

Personal Insights: A Self-Examination Kit for Women *can be ordered through* Hysteria. *See page 110 for details.*

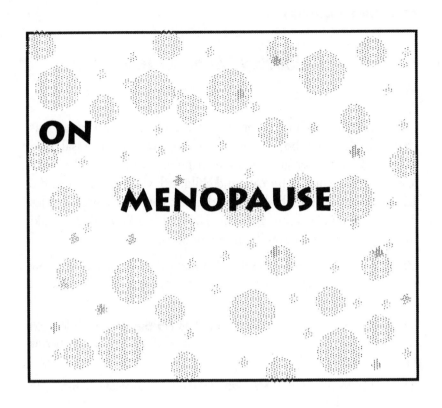

ON MENOPAUSE

Celebrity Menopause
by Mary-Lou Weisman

On the Brink of Menopause
by Effin Older

Menoprom
by Jude McGee

Celebrity Menopause

by Mary-Lou Weisman

Menopause is hot. Hot flashes are cool. The change has changed. Now everybody wants to climb onto the menopausal band wagon. Hot flashes are observed in public with a wonder once reserved for the aurora borealis and childbirth videos. Not since the 12-Step Program and the Betty Ford Clinic have so many celebrities rushed to confess. Here are some tabloid headlines that should show up on your newsstand any day now.

LIZ TAYLOR: "Menopause Nearly Killed Me." The plucky star tells how an overdose of estrogen replacement therapy triggered a deadly attack of faux PMS.

SHIRLEY MACLAINE: "The Last One Was No Sweat." Middle aged actress and pro-former-life activist says she suffered no hot flashes as Egyptian princess.

"I had GLORIA STEINEM'S Menopause" reveals change-of-life surrogate Mary Beth Whitehead.

"I Never Had It. Neither Did Jim." JAN MORRIS, sex change author, explodes myth of male menopause.

PATTI DAVIS signs contract for new book: ***Mom, Menopause and Me.***

"I Grew Up Too Fast." Breaking a 30-year silence, a tough but teary ROSEANNE BARR talks candidly about her early childhood menopause.

"It's all a male plot to keep women looking young and attractive." GERMAINE GREER says no to estrogen replacement therapy.

"Menstrual Daughters of Menopausal Mothers" 12-step, self-help group forms.

MADONNA stars in made-for-menopause video, **"Can't Wait to Get Hot All Over."**

On the Brink of Menopause

by Effin Older

For my 50th birthday my daughter gave me an easy-to-apply, lasts-for-days, temporary tattoo. She dares me to wear it where everyone can see it.

She also gave me Gail Sheehy's book, *The Silent Passage*.

I haven't applied the tattoo yet, but I've read the Sheehy book from cover to cover. I had wanted to read it ever since I missed my period for the first time. That was a momentous occasion. After 38 years of being as regular as my grandmother's afternoon cup of tea, I was now either pregnant at 50 ... or on the brink of menopause.

Like many women of my generation, my mother never discussed menopause with me; in fact, she never discussed anything related to bodies or sex. So it was with trepidation that, a few months before my 50th birthday, I decided to bring up the subject of menopause.

I called her, thinking it would be easier (on both of us) to talk by phone. I came straight out with it. "Ma, I want to talk to you about menopause."

Silence. Then, "What do you want to talk about *that* for?"

"Because I've been reading a lot about it lately, and one thing I've read is that a daughter's menopause is often similar to her mother's. So I wanted to know what yours was like."

More silence.

The conversation was only a minute old and already I was fidgeting. I was wishing I could hang up when she said, "Just like everybody else's, I suppose." Her tone, flat and dismissive, signaled me to drop the subject. I plowed on.

"But, Ma, is that all you can tell me? I mean, didn't you have hot flashes or night sweats or anything?"

She sighed again, this time heavily. "How come, all of a sudden, hot flashes are so popular?"

"Don't you think it's about time?"

"Well, no one ever talked to *me* about it." Then she added, "And probably that's the way it should be."

I said quietly, "I guess times have changed." I couldn't press her further. It would have been nice to share this intimacy with my mother, but I was losing my resolve. "Oh, well, I guess I'll just have to read more books and wait and see what happens."

There was a long quietness on both ends of the phone. Then, as I was about to hang up, my 76-year-old mother started talking. And talking and talking. She described five years of hot flashes that always seemed to happen in public places, night sweats that left her drenched, and a constant feeling of irritability. She said she hadn't known if what she was going through was normal or crazy. "All I had to read was a couple of those home-medicine, marriage-guide books that you could order through the mail. There was no what's-her-name — the woman who wrote that book — in my time."

"Sheehy," I filled in.

When I hung up an hour later, my curiosity about my mother's menopause had been satisfied; whether my menopause pattern will fit hers remains to be seen.

But in the meantime, I was now filled with a new curiosity. What had my mother read in those "home-medicine, marriage-guide books that you could order through the mail"? Who were the Gail Sheehys of *her* day? My mother couldn't remember the authors of the books she'd read, but after spending several hours the following day in the library thumbing through volumes of marriage guides, I was certain one of them would have been T.H. Van de Velde, M.D.

Dr. Van de Velde was one of the most influential, widely read and highly praised authors of marriage guides. His book, *Ideal Marriage*, was first published in 1928 but was still in print — in its 39th edition — in 1962.

Here is Van de Velde on menopause: "Caprice, excitability, increased impulsiveness combined with diminished powers of reason and reflection ... the change can cause a degree of psychic suffering and storm which is positively DANGEROUS [sic] to themselves and others."

Diminished powers of reason? Psychic suffering? DANGER? These were hardly sentiments designed to reassure my mother that the change she was undergoing was natural, temporary, and not to be feared. It's no wonder she didn't want to talk about it.

In 1929, one year after *Ideal Marriage,* Dr. Joseph Tenenbaum published *The Riddle of Sex.* After Van de Velde, my mother must have looked forward with great anticipation to Tenenbaum. I can only imagine how great was her despair when she opened its cover.

Here's Tenenbaum on menopause: "Climacteric ... marks a new era of existence. The fountain of youth has been exhausted ... signs of decline are beginning to appear .... The climacteric female acquires coarser features, a coarser voice and ... may grow a beard and mustache.

"Women, who formerly may have been of an agreeable disposition, become restless, irritable, angry and easily inflammable, ... hesitant, moody and capricious."

As if all this weren't bad enough, Tenenbaum goes on to say, "Stout believers ... may suddenly become sex mad. The former church devotee may now turn out to be a devilish Bacchante. Such a woman ... is a source of ridicule to others and a riddle to herself."

I closed *The Riddle of Sex* and tried to imagine my churchgoing, roly-poly, 5-foot-2-inch, bread-making Mom attempting to seduce another member of the Brownington Congregational Church with her husky voice, beard, and mustache!

It was the likes of Van de Velde and Tenenbaum who kept up the myth of menopausal madness, and whom I can thank, at least in part, for my mother's reluctance to talk about her change of life.

Luckily, over the years, attitudes changed.

In 1972, Alex Comfort in *The Joy of Sex* wrote that "the various and absurd opinions relative to the ceasing of the menstrual discharge ... have tended to embitter the hours of many a sensible woman ... and some practitioners seem not to have endeavored to correct them with the diligence and humanity which such an object requires."

Amen.

Shere Hite in the 1977 *Hite Report* asked women themselves how age affected their lives, especially their desire for sex. Did it increase or decrease with age? Two women responded thus:

"I didn't know getting older would make sex better! I'm 51 now and just getting started."

"I'm post-menopausal. I enjoy sex more since I no longer fear pregnancy. Because I enjoy it more, so does my husband. He finds it a pleasant surprise … in fact, I put the excitement in his life!"

These responses were a far cry from the picture of the menopausal woman — capricious, depressed, sex-mad and bearded — drawn by Van de Velde and Tenenbaum. It seemed that, with the publication of *The Hite Report*, at last the menopausal woman was out of their clutches.

I don't plan to write a book about menopause, but I feel I can make a small but significant contribution to women the world over in another way. It's about this problem of night sweats. They haven't hit me yet, but when they do, I'll be ready. You see, I've designed a secret weapon. I got the idea from a sportswear catalogue featuring those new-age fabrics that allow you to sweat without getting wet. Through some miracle, the sweat gets sucked ("wicked" is the technical term) away from your body, out through the fabric and into the air, all the while keeping your body as dry as a piece of yesterday's toast.

So here it is, my solution for night sweats.

A wicking nightie.

Perhaps Anne Klein can come up with a sexy design.

Meanwhile, I still have the tattoo, and I think I'll take my daughter's dare. That low-cut, sleeveless, black satin dress is the number I'll wear it with — on my right arm, just below my shoulder.

❖

Menoprom

by Jude McGee

Pundits agree, as the big bulge of baby boomers hits middle age with both feet running, it is an absolute priority to come up with a fitting expression of our individual and collective glee. Women want to kick up their heels and celebrate the new life that is possible once they have achieved the state Margaret Mead calls "post-menopausal zest." And we need a special celebration. After all, the achievements of the first part of our lives, saddled as we were with everyone else's ideas about who we should be, are tremendous. Better, however, is the anticipation of the glories to come.

To wit, and brevity is ever: no more pharmaceutical devices and jellies to prevent babies; no more being stared at as if one were an exhibit. But the best thing is — and Carolyn Heilbrun said it best in *Writing a Woman's Life* — no longer living a story someone else wrote. After menopause, we can write our own stories. This is a joyous, magnificent, giddy-making occasion; it needs its own very special celebration, with the right combination of pomp and circumstance, yet where a whoopee cushion would not be out of place. And I have it!

The Menoprom

At the Menoprom, we can literally kick up our heels and dance with whomever we like, having made sure to have invited all the people this would include. At the Menoprom, there will be no limiting ourselves to only one date, and for sure each and every one of us will have met and retained the friendship of many elegantly suitable dance partners, be they sons, lovers, galloping galfriends, dykes on bikes (invite the bikes, too), one of our series of husbands, or one of our serially monogamous mates.

As second-wave feminists, since we've been taking the heat for it anyway, we could stage events celebrated in the male media myth, like a bra burning.

And clothes. We could really show the world the capabilities of a mature imagination. Tulle with Doc Martens, indeed! How passé and boring compared to what we, postmenopausal zesty, will come up with! What menoprommer does not have a fecund brain waiting in the wings now that the fecund uterus is done?

The Menoprom will combine the joy, anticipation, tension, and respect that is required of the important moment when we pause, not from men, but from being mom. Celebrating momopause just as we celebrated, in a sense, the beginning of adulthood with a gala, terrifying, competitive party of parties. Remember the joys and horrors of the senior prom? Well how about a prom for seniors of another sort — we who have no more periods and sing to no one else's tune. So what if it's because they ignore us; we have learned we are enough to satisfy ourselves. Right!

The Menoprom with all the memories of our first prom to guide us, and upon which we can improve! Do it again with all the knowledge of hindsight? I don't think so! Remember when we had to get the right guy (or at least the right type of guy) to take us, and we'd hide out to avoid the geeks and pine for the sports heroes or dead-poets-society hopefuls? Well, for the Menoprom, that would not have to happen. First of all, for the Menoprom, we do the inviting! And it can be anyone. It is unlikely that in our four or five decades on the planet we have not bred a son or married at least one dazzler, and we are not limited to the opposite sex or any specific age group! Everyone will have the perfect prom date! Lots of shrinks tell us of the efficacy of rewriting history; here we can do that and party, too. All that may have eluded us as teens can now be experienced in later life, when we are conscious enough to truly enjoy it.

We take what we like from the past and forget the rest.

Hair

This is great, because my actual prom hairdo made me look older than I will probably ever look in real life, so I can try for a facsimile — or any do in between— not to mention any color! Remember when the only colors were black, brown, and blonde, with the latter highly stigmatized as "bottle"except for a Nordic few? Now who among us would confess to the prosaism of not coloring, and hennas are just the tip.

Decorations

They were of true importance at the old prom, and now that we have cast embarrassment to the wind, we can cast all our embarrassing items around the hall: tampons with the strings cheerfully waving, stockings, garter belts, all those early report cards we hid from the boys because we did so much better in school.

Music

We all confess to inexplicable fondness for the songs that accompanied our deepest anguish, and what was more anguishing than our teens? The Menoprom will give a new and joyous setting to those old tunes! And we'll bring on the new ones, too. Invite Killer Bikini, Sweet Honey in the Rock, everyone from the Ladyslipper Catalog, Queen Ida, and the Women's Philharmonic.

We baby boomers are a big enough group for a critical mass, and the time for action is now. Celebrate the hell out of that milestone of milestones in a woman's life, menopause.

LET YOUR FINGERS DO THE WALKING: ONE STOP SHOPPING FOR THE FEMALE CONSUMER

A selection of
books and miscellaneous
available as a service
to our readers
directly from Hysteria.

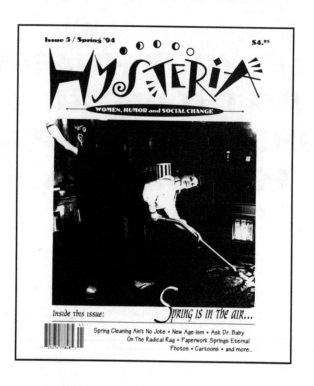

GET THE LAST LAUGH WITH *HYSTERIA*,
THE HUMOR MAGAZINE FOR THE '90s WOMAN.

"Irreverent, insightful, brash and sometimes bawdy."
—*New York Newsday*

"Comics, totally loony archive photos, general silliness, feminism, and frazzle. Check it out."

—*WomanZine*

$18.00 FOR ONE YEAR (4 ISSUES)
$4.95 FOR A SAMPLE COPY
SEND CHECK OR MONEY ORDER TO:
HYSTERIA BOX 8581 BREWSTER STATION BRIDGEPORT, CT 06605

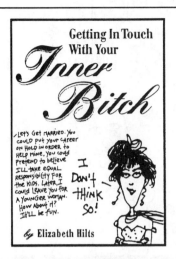

Getting In Touch With Your Inner Bitch
by Elizabeth Hilts

There is an integral, powerful part of each of us which is going unrecognized. It is the Inner Bitch. Don't even pretend you don't know what I'm talking about. The Inner Bitch is the Bette Davis in each of us, walking around with a cigarette in one hand, a martini in the other, calling a dump a dump. The Inner Bitch calls it as she sees it.

For the woman who wants to laugh out loud and speak her mind, *Getting In Touch With Your Inner Bitch* is the ultimate book.

Hysteria Publications, paperback
$7.95 + $1.00 s/h

CT residents add 6% sales tax
Send check or money order to:
Hysteria
PO Box 8581, Brewster Station
Bridgeport, CT 06605

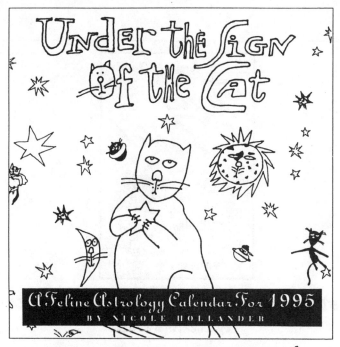

Under the Sign of the Cat
A Feline Astrology Calendar for 1995
by Nicole Hollander

Humankind has been wondering for centuries about the mysteries of cats: How can they have such small brains and such large personalities?

It took Nicole Hollander, famed for her Sylvia cartoon strip, to make the connection between the inscrutable feline and the heavenly spheres.

You don't have to be a cat lover to find this one of the funniest cartoon calendars you've ever seen!

16-month Cartoon Wall Calendar   12" x 24" (open)

$12.95 plus $1.50 s/h

(CT residents add 6% sales tax)

SEND CHECK OR MONEY ORDER TO:

HYSTERIA BOX 8581 BREWSTER STATION BRIDGEPORT, CT 06605

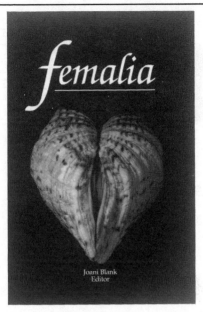

Femalia

As a leader of women's sexuality workshops, Joani Blank found that most women believe their genitals are not quite normal, let alone attractive or beautiful. These 32 photographs of women's vulvas, strikingly different in shape, color, and proportion, prove otherwise.

Femalia, edited by Joani Blank, is a groundbreaking book — informative and beautiful.

"...a magic mirror..." — Annie Sprinkle

Down There Press, paperback
$14.50 + $1.00 s/h

CT residents add 6% sales tax
Send check or money order to:
Hysteria
PO Box 8581, Brewster Station
Bridgeport, CT 06605

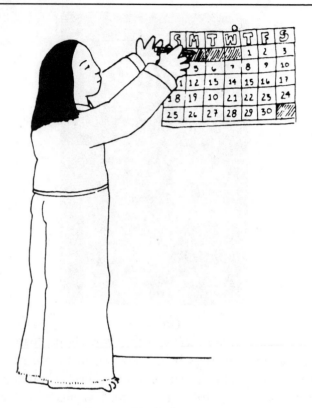

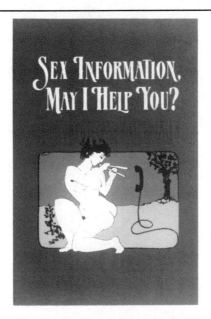

Sex Information, May I Help You?

Fascinating and educational. An entertaining saga of San Francisco Sex Information switchboard volunteers and their callers. Covering a lot of topics, including sexually transmitted diseases, sexual turn-ons, group sex, masturbation, pregnancy, contraception, disability, aging, cross-dressing, and more.

"…an excellent model on how to speak directly about sex…." *San Francisco Chronicle*

Down There Press, paperback
$9.50 + $1.00 s/h

CT residents add 6% sales tax
Send check or money order to:
Hysteria
PO Box 8581, Brewster Station
Bridgeport, CT 06605

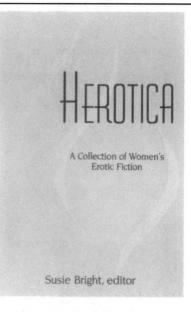

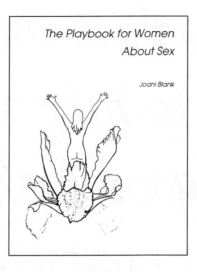

The Playbook for Women About Sex
Joani Blank

The Playbook for Women About Sex

A sensible course in self-awareness, encouraging the reader to understand his/her sexual history, body image, partner choices, turn-ons, and communication patterns. Casual and reassuring.

"…a fun approach to sexual self-awareness…."
SIECCAN

Down There Press, paperback
$4.50 + $1.00 s/h

CT residents add 6% sales tax
Send check or money order to:
Hysteria
PO Box 8581, Brewster Station
Bridgeport, CT 06605

Isn't it time to take a good look at yourself?

Personal Insights

A self-examination kit for women, designed by Dr. Debra Gussman (see page 87 above). A detailed instruction manual guides you through a safe, easy, genital self-examination in the privacy of your home. Contains a light, a specially designed mirror, and a speculum.

"…today's woman wants to see for herself.…"
Nexus

Debra Gussman, M.D., kit
$24.99 + $4.00 s/h

CT residents add 6% sales tax
Send check or money order to:
Hysteria
PO Box 8581, Brewster Station
Bridgeport, CT 06605

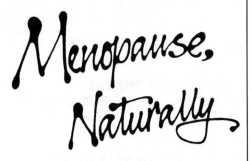

PREPARING FOR THE SECOND HALF OF LIFE

Sadja Greenwood, M.D.

Illustrations by Marcia Quackenbush

Menopause Naturally

This book addresses all the questions women have about menopause and the conflicting information they hear.

Includes guidance on screening tests for osteoporosis, non-hormonal treatments, new ways to deal with hot flashes, what natural progesterone is, testosterone therapy, exercise, diet, and how to maintain postmenopausal zest.

"…unique, common sense guide for every woman…"
Gloria Steinem

Volcano Press, paperback
$13.95 + $1.00 s/h

CT residents add 6% sales tax
Send check or money order to:
Hysteria
PO Box 8581 Brewster Station
Bridgeport, CT 06605

ORDER FORM

HYSTERIA: THE WOMEN'S HUMOR MAGAZINE

_____ **ONE YEAR SUBSCRIPTION (4 ISSUES) $18.00**
_____ **SAMPLE ISSUE $4.95**

GETTING IN TOUCH WITH YOUR INNER BITCH $7.95
BY ELIZABETH HILTS

UNDER THE SIGN OF THE CAT: $12.95
A FELINE ASTROLOGY CALENDAR FOR 1995
BY NICOLE HOLLANDER

AT YOUR FINGERTIPS: $7.95
THE CARE & MAINTENANCE OF A VAGINA

FEMALIA $14.50
EDITED BY JOANI BLANK

PERIOD. $9.95

SEX INFORMATION, MAY I HELP YOU? $9.50

HEROTICA: A COLLECTION OF $8.50
WOMEN'S EROTIC FICTION

THE PLAYBOOK FOR WOMEN ABOUT SEX $4.50

PERSONAL INSIGHTS: $24.99
A SELF-EXAM KIT FOR WOMEN

MENOPAUSE NATURALLY $13.95

ADD $1.00 PER TITLE FOR SHIPPING/HANDLING
CT RESIDENTS ADD 6% SALES TAX
(EXCEPT FOR HYSTERIA SUBSCRIPTION)

ENCLOSED IS MY CHECK OR MONEY ORDER FOR:

NAME:

ADDRESS:

CITY/STATE/ZIP:

HYSTERIA
BOX 8581 BRIDGEPORT, CT 06605 · (203) 333-9399